Information Circular 9502

Guidelines for the Prediction and Control of Methane Emissions on Longwalls

By Steven J. Schatzel, Ph.D., C. Özgen Karacan, Ph.D., Robert B. Krog, Gabriel S. Esterhuizen, Ph.D., and Gerrit V. R. Goodman, Ph.D.

DEPARTMENT OF HEALTH AND HUMAN SERVICES
Centers for Disease Control and Prevention
National Institute for Occupational Safety and Health
Pittsburgh Research Laboratory
Pittsburgh, PA

March 2008

Disclaimer

Mention of any company or product does not constitute endorsement by the National Institute for Occupational Safety and Health (NIOSH). In addition, citations to Web sites external to NIOSH do not constitute NIOSH endorsement of the sponsoring organizations or their programs or products. Furthermore, NIOSH is not responsible for the content of these Web sites.

Ordering Information

To receive documents or other information about occupational safety and health topics, contact NIOSH at

> Telephone: **1–800–CDC–INFO** (1–800–232–4636)
> TTY: 1–888–232–6348
> e-mail: cdcinfo@cdc.gov
>
> or visit the NIOSH Web site at **www.cdc.gov/niosh**.

For a monthly update on news at NIOSH, subscribe to NIOSH *eNews* by visiting **www.cdc.gov/niosh/eNews**.

DHHS (NIOSH) Publication No. 2008–114

March 2008

SAFER • HEALTHIER • PEOPLE™

CONTENTS

CONTENTS—Continued

ILLUSTRATIONS

CONTENTS—Continued

CONTENTS—Continued

TABLES

Page

ACRONYMS AND ABBREVIATIONS USED IN THIS REPORT

BH	borehole
BME	borehole monitoring experiment
CH_4	methane
FLAC	Fast Lagrangian Analysis of Continua
GEM	Generalized Equation-of-State Model
GGV	gob gas venthole
H–T	head-to-tail
NIOSH	National Institute for Occupational Safety and Health
PRL	Pittsburgh Research Laboratory (NIOSH)
PVC	polyvinyl chloride
T–H	tail-to-head
USBM	U.S. Bureau of Mines

UNIT OF MEASURE ABBREVIATIONS USED IN THIS REPORT

cc/g	cubic centimeter per gram
cfm	cubic foot per minute
cm/s	centimeter per second
cps	counts per second
ft	foot
ft^3	cubic foot
ft/day	foot per day
ft/min	foot per minute
g/cc	gram per cubic centimeter
in	inch
in/s	inch per second
kPa	kilopascal
m	meter
m/day	meter per day
m/min	meter per minute
m/s	meter per second
m^3	cubic meter
m^3/day	cubic meter per day
m^3/min	cubic meter per minute
m^3/s	cubic meter per second
md	millidarcy
min	minute
MMscf	million standard cubic feet
Pa	pascal
psi	pound-force per square inch
psia	pound-force per square inch absolute
scf	standard cubic feet
scf/day	standard cubic feet per day
scf/ton	standard cubic feet per ton
sec	second

GUIDELINES FOR THE PREDICTION AND CONTROL OF METHANE EMISSIONS ON LONGWALLS

By Steven J. Schatzel, Ph.D.,[1] C. Özgen Karacan, Ph.D.,[2] Robert B. Krog,[3] Gabriel S. Esterhuizen, Ph.D.,[2] and Gerrit V. R. Goodman, Ph.D.[4]

EXECUTIVE SUMMARY

Although longwall mining productivity can far exceed that of room-and-pillar mining, the total methane emissions per extracted volume associated with longwall sections are generally higher than those for continuous miner or pillar removal sections. Increased face advance rates, increased productivities, increased panel sizes, and more extensive gate road developments have challenged existing designs for controlling methane on longwalls.

Methane control research by the National Institute for Occupational Safety and Health (NIOSH) recently examined a number of practices designed to maintain concentrations in mine air within statutory limits and consistently below the lower explosive limit. These included a reservoir modeling approach to predict methane inflows in gate road entries. The outputs suggested that emission rates in the gate roads decreased with the use of shielding boreholes and increased degasification time. Also, mining perpendicular to the face cleats liberated more gas into the mine workings, emissions were almost a linear function of Langmuir pressure and volume, and emissions were inversely related to sorption time constant.

Subsequent simulations predicted changes in methane drainage using in-seam boreholes. The results showed that longer degasification times resulted in lower face emission rates. Premining degasification produced more methane than that produced during panel extraction, a fact attributed to the already decreased methane content of the coalbed. This work concluded that longer premining degasification periods would be more advantageous to the operator.

The industry trend toward increasing longwall face width can produce increased methane emissions from the face due to a higher volume of cut coal on the face conveyor. Two methods were used to estimate face methane levels on longer faces. In the first method, segmented methane data were extrapolated for greater face widths. The second method estimated emissions contributions from the shearer, face conveyor, panel belt, longwall face, and ribs, and summed these for wider panels.

Permeability changes in the gob behind the longwall shields were estimated using a NIOSH-developed numerical model. The results showed that permeability was highest near the edges and corners of the gob.

---

[1]Lead research geologist.
[2]Senior service fellow.
[3]Associate service fellow.
[4]Team leader, Ventilation and Explosion Prevention Group, Disaster Prevention and Response Branch.
Pittsburgh Research Laboratory, National Institute for Occupational Safety and Health, Pittsburgh, PA.

Gob gas ventholes (GGVs) represent a very effective means for controlling methane gas on longwall faces. NIOSH work showed that (1) larger-diameter GGVs produced more methane, but at the expense of increased dilution due to the presence of mine ventilation air in the boreholes; (2) GGVs should not be sunk into the caved zone of a longwall panel since more ventilation airflow will be sent to the boreholes; and (3) increased slotted casing lengths improved GGV production.

NIOSH conducted an extensive borehole monitoring experiment (BME) to assess the impacts of longwall mining on development of the coalbed reservoir. Three boreholes were drilled to different stratigraphic horizons in advance of undermining by a longwall and instrumented to measure pre- and postmining in situ permeabilities and gas pressures. The data showed that mining-induced disturbances occurred 20–46 m (80–150 ft) ahead of the retreating longwall face, causing a corresponding increase in formation permeability.

In this report, several practical guidelines are recommended for controlling longwall coalbed methane. All predictions are based on determinations made for the Pittsburgh Coalbed in southwestern Pennsylvania.

- It is recommended to use shielding degasification boreholes to decrease emission rates by at least 25% for development entries. Drill these boreholes as close as practically possible (~27 m (90 ft)) to the entries and operate them for at least 6 months to achieve a 25%–50% decrease in emission rates (Section 1).

- Equations for predicting methane emissions rates into gate road developments are presented in Table 3 (Section 1). These relationships assume a supercritical longwall panel developed in the Pittsburgh Coalbed.

- For a longwall panel width greater than 305 m (1,000 ft), a trilateral borehole configuration is recommended for effective draining of methane. Short across-panel holes at close spacing can also be effective in degassing a panel. The required number of holes will depend on seam anisotropic reservoir conditions, but at least 12 holes for a 3,400-m (11,000-ft) long panel are recommended to achieve the same degasification as the trilateral configuration (Section 2).

- If less than 12 months are available for premining gas drainage, it is recommended that degasification be continued until the borehole is approached by mining. This approach maximizes the quantity of removed methane and reduces methane emission rates (Section 2).

- To avoid shearer coal production delays, it is recommended that continuous GGV production be assured while GGVs are within about 500 ft of the working face. In many mines, the quantity of coalbed methane removed by a GGV is potentially 75% of the volume of gas emissions on the longwall face. A similar finding was observed by prior NIOSH research. If an operating GGV ceases producing gas, the gas that was being removed will enter the ventilation system (Section 3).

- Assuming a well-caved gob, increasing the longwall face length by X% will increase the rate of methane emissions by, at most, two-thirds of X% (Section 4).

- The length of the slotted casing section of a GGV will strongly influence its level of gas production. To effectively design the slotted casing section of a GGV, it is recommended to:
  - Review the local geology to identify the location of gas-bearing units; and
  - Set the top of the slotted section at the highest gas-producing stratigraphic horizon (Section 6).

- Completing a GGV into the caved zone is counterproductive and increases the likelihood of intermittent production from increased-width, supercritical panels. Therefore, the completion depth of GGVs should be at least 14 m (45 ft) above the top of coal for longwall panels, particularly in the Northern Appalachian Basin (Sections 6 and 7).

- Emphasize continuous GGV production since it will potentially produce 40%–50% more coalbed gas than GGVs operating intermittently (Section 7).

- Increasing the longwall panel width increases the quantity of methane present because of the increased fractured reservoir volume. However, this increase does not enhance the performance of GGVs. As panel width increases, the effectiveness of GGVs completed near the tailgate margin will not extend as close to the headgate side. Drilling GGVs on the headgate side or near the panel centerline can produce coalbed gas from this portion of the panel (Sections 5 and 7).

- In favorable cases, GGVs drilled on the headgate side can be effective. Completion depths must isolate the borehole from communication with the ventilation network. These findings are based on supercritical panel designs (Section 7).

- Mining-induced fracturing was observed to occur 24–46 m (80–150 ft) ahead of the mine face. Boreholes and exhausters should be installed before this occurs (Section 8).

- Data were reviewed for GGV configurations completed from 7 to 32 m (24 to 106 ft) above the mined coalbed for supercritical panels in the Northern Appalachian Basin. It is recommended that GGVs be completed toward the top of this interval and be designed to include the Sewickley Coalbed. Permeability increases following undermining were dramatic, with increases of about 100–500 times the premining values and instantaneous increases of up to about 1,000 times these values. These measurements did not differ significantly despite differences in borehole configurations. Fracture permeability pathways remain high to the mined coalbed toward the top of the described interval, yet the likelihood of drawing ventilation air into the borehole is minimized (Section 8).

ACKNOWLEDGMENTS

The authors thank Thomas P. Mucho, W. P. Diamond, and Fred Garcia, all retired from NIOSH, for their significant contributions to the completion of the technical work throughout this research project. The authors acknowledge the valuable technical and editorial input received from field reviewers Pramod C. Thakur, Ph.D., CONSOL Energy, Inc.; Jerry C. Tien, Ph.D., University of Missouri-Rolla; and Thomas McNider, Jim Walter Resources, Inc. The authors also acknowledge Robert J. Tuchman, Technical Writer-Editor, Centers for Disease Control and Prevention, and Joe Schall, the Giles Writer-in-Residence at The Pennsylvania State University, for their substantial contributions to improving the clarity and quality of this report. In addition, the authors thank the cooperating mine operators and staff who made these research efforts possible and who have requested anonymity.

BACKGROUND

In today's competitive energy market, U.S. deep coal mine producers often choose longwall over room-and-pillar mining because of the high productivities and improved safety benefits that can be achieved. The longwall mining method requires an adequate and suitable coal reserve where the coal is of good quality and where geologic conditions are appropriate. Because of the nature of longwall mining, total methane emissions associated with longwall mining are generally higher for a specific volume of mined coal than for continuous miner or pillar removal sections. During longwall mining, a large block of coal is extracted and the immediate roof, three to six times the thickness of the mined coalbed, extensively fractures and falls into the mine void [Singh and Kendorski 1981; Palchik 2003]. The stress relief in the surrounding strata that results from this caving creates large horizontal fractures along bedding planes and vertical fractures in the strata overlying and underlying the caved zone. These mining-induced fractures provide extensive pathways for gas migration from the surrounding coalbeds and other gas-bearing strata into the mining environment. The fractured zone is present in the roof and floor can vary up to 100 times the height of the mined coalbed of the overburden [Curl 1978; Thakur 1981] depending on the mechanical properties of the rock layers, thickness of the overburden, and size of the panel.

The methane that originates and accumulates in the gob above the mined-out panel is the main source of methane emissions during longwall mining. Prior monitoring studies directed at longwall face emissions indicate that only a small portion of the overall methane emission and gas production is emitted at the mine face [Tauziede et al. 1997; Diamond and Garcia 1999]. It has been reported that methane contributions from the subsided strata (gob) generally account for 80%–94% of the methane present in the ventilation system of an operating longwall [Curl 1978; Schatzel et al. 1992]. These research findings suggest that typical longwall face emissions account for no more than 20% of longwall emissions and as little as 6% of the total emissions at one site [Schatzel et al. 1992] and potentially less at very gassy mines. However, this particular emissions source can be critical in relation to underground safety. Face areas on longwall mining sections present specific challenges for methane control techniques where high production rates can cause relatively high methane emission rates, making it difficult to meet statutory limits on methane concentrations at face and tailgate sampling locations. Recent input from NIOSH stakeholders suggests that the longwall tailgate T-junction area is crucial for effective ventilation air dilution of methane emissions and will be a subject of upcoming research.

Available methane control systems have been challenged by recent developments in longwall mining. These developments include increased face advance rates leading to increased coal production, increased longwall panel sizes resulting in more extensive gate road developments, and the generally deeper and gassier workings of U.S. coal mines. All of these have presented additional challenges for longwall face ventilation. Work by Diamond and Garcia [1999] reported the predicted impact of face extensions at two longwall operations in the Pocahontas Coalbed from mining operations in northwestern Virginia. Increasing face length from 229 to 305 m (750 to 1,000 ft) (33%) led to a predicted increase in face methane emissions from 8.0 to 8.6 m^3/min (280 to 300 cfm), or an increase of about 7%. At an adjoining operation, a similar increase in face width led to a predicted methane emissions increase of about 13%, from 14.2 to 16.1 m^3/min (502 to 567 cfm). Variabilities in mine design and methane control practices between the two mine sites were the primary causes of the different predicted methane emission rates for the 1,000-ft face widths. Schatzel et al. [2006] and Krog et al. [2006] produced empirical models of methane emissions for longer longwall faces for a mine operating in the Pittsburgh Coalbed of southwestern Pennsylvania. The calculated methane emissions by Krog et al. were determined on the basis of 61-m (200-ft) increment increases in face length. Peak methane emissions increased from 6.6 to 9.1 m^3/min (234 to 322 cfm), or 38%, as face length increased from roughly 305 to 488 m (1,000 to 1,600 ft). This determination was based on computed constants associated with specified methane sources (shearer, face conveyor, belt conveyor, background emissions from the coal face, and background emissions from the adjoining ribs in the intake gate roads) and a zero time delay "idealized" longwall face pass of the shearer. Schatzel et al. [2006] predicted methane emissions on longer longwall faces for lengths of 366, 427, and 488 m (1,200, 1,400, and 1,600 ft) of 5.4, 6.4, and 7.4 m^3/min (191, 225, and 263 cfm), increases of 36%, 61%, and 88%, respectively, over the base case. The lower face emission rates predicted by Schatzel et al. compared to those of Krog et al. arose from the inclusion of production delays and average emission rates in the first study compared to no delays and peak emission rates in the second study.

The increasing coal productivities from longwall operations have led to greater volumes of coalbed methane gas entering the underground mine environments from exposed coal surfaces and from cut coal on the conveyor belting. Production advances in longwall mining have significantly challenged currently available methane control designs for reducing the potential for methane explosions. Such designs require that reservoir pressures and gas contents be reduced to limit migration of coalbed gas into the mine atmosphere, and these techniques require sufficient lead time to achieve sufficient reductions in methane inflow. Coalbed methane emission rates can vary widely among different coalbeds and should be considered in the application of the recommendations provided. Even within the same coalbed, geographic changes can produce changes to gas storage or emission-related geotechnical parameters, thereby modifying coalbed methane emission behavior.

1. RESERVOIR MODELING FOR PREDICTING METHANE EMISSIONS IN DEVELOPMENT HEADINGS (ENTRIES)

Overview

Planning, designing, and optimizing ventilation are important steps to eliminate any accumulation of explosive methane-air mixtures in the development and extraction phases of longwall coal mining. Insufficient ventilation and unexpectedly high methane liberation rates can overwhelm the existing ventilation capacity and result in elevated concentrations of methane gas, which can lead to production interruptions and endanger the safety of workers underground. Mine operators usually try to supply maximum ventilation air based on the capacity of the system and the predicted needs underground. However, ventilation capacity may decrease over time due to leakage, especially as the gate road entries get longer. Also, increased mining advance rates and changes in geologic conditions can produce substantial increases in methane emission rates that can challenge and overwhelm ventilation system designs. Consequently, it has become increasingly difficult to keep methane levels under statutory limits by ventilation alone, and ventilation requirements may depart significantly from initially planned values. This condition can both limit the advance of a particular section and increase the risk for an ignition or explosion. Thus, it is important to develop an understanding of key parameters influencing methane emission rates and sound techniques to optimize mine ventilation and methane drainage effectiveness to ensure a safer work environment.

One key requirement in meeting this objective is the ability to predict methane emission rates. For gate road developments of longwall panels, the prediction of methane emission rates is affected by both mining parameters and coalbed reservoir parameters. Although changes made to mining parameters, such as development rate and gate road length, can impact methane inflow, similar options do not exist when dealing with coalbed reservoir properties, such as coalbed thickness and reservoir pressure. Thus, it is important to understand the effects of these parameters on methane inflow rates in order to be able to control methane emissions effectively.

When it is difficult to keep methane under statutory limits by ventilation alone, one of the most effective approaches is to drill horizontal boreholes in the coalbed to drain excessive methane before mining starts [Brunner et al. 1997; Noack 1998]. Effective horizontal methane drainage well designs were pioneered by the U.S. Bureau of Mines (USBM) and by CONSOL Energy in the 1970s [Cervik et al. 1975; Thakur and Poundstone 1980; Prosser et al. 1981; Diamond 1994; Thakur 2006]. In-seam horizontal wells drilled into the planned longwall panels and ahead of development mining serve two purposes. First, wells reduce the methane content of the coalbed in and around the panel area where development mining will be conducted. Second, wells shield the developing entries from methane migration from the coalbed surrounding the roadways. This approach has been shown to be effective in reducing methane emission rates. Thakur [2006] discussed methane drainage methods where the borehole drilling trailed gate road development, but was in advance of the longwall face. Prior research that reported horizontal well performance comprised novel studies, but generally used empirical relationships [Cervik et al. 1975; Thakur and Poundstone 1980; Diamond 1994]. Thus, an engineering-based analytical approach was proposed to develop horizontal borehole design improvements to enhance the methane control and ventilation system.

A reservoir model was configured to calculate methane emission rates during development mining [Karacan, forthcoming; Karacan et al. 2007a]. The model included a three-entry tailgate and headgate development layout, which is typical of coal mines operating in Pittsburgh Coalbed in the southwestern Pennsylvania section of the Northern Appalachian Basin (Figure 1).

During the mining of headgate and tailgate entries of the study mine, ventilation air qualities and methane in flow rates were measured by the operating mining company using methanometers and anemometers at the monitoring locations shown in Figure 1. Methane inflow rates were quantified based on the measured data. The data were reported as average monthly concentrations of methane, airflow rate, raw and clean tonnages of produced coal, and total linear distances advanced during mining. The length of each entry section was around 3,350 m (11,000 ft) and required 8–9 months to mine.

The in-mine measurements of methane inflows were matched with the model predictions to calibrate the reservoir model. Various models were developed to investigate methane emissions during development mining by relating mining parameters (Table 1) and coalbed reservoir parameters (Table 2). In the first set of analyses, the effects of mining parameters with and without horizontal degasification wellbores were investigated by keeping the coalbed reservoir parameters at their base levels (Table 2) while varying the mining parameters (Table 1). In the second set of analyses, mining rate was kept constant and coalbed reservoir parameters were varied to investigate the effects of these parameters on methane emissions (Table 2).

The methane concentrations reported in Table 1 represent values for the last open crosscut within development gate roads. The cleat permeability and effective porosity data shown in Table 2 represent values for the Pittsburgh Coalbed in southwestern Pennsylvania and may vary from determinations made for other locations within the coalbed. The values given for shielding well distances to development entries were used to show trends in borehole effectiveness for reducing emissions in relation to entry proximity. In practice, drilling a borehole 5.8 m (19 ft) from a development entry would create a range of operational challenges. Mine operators typically drill methane drainage boreholes 15–46 m (50–150) ft from development entries.

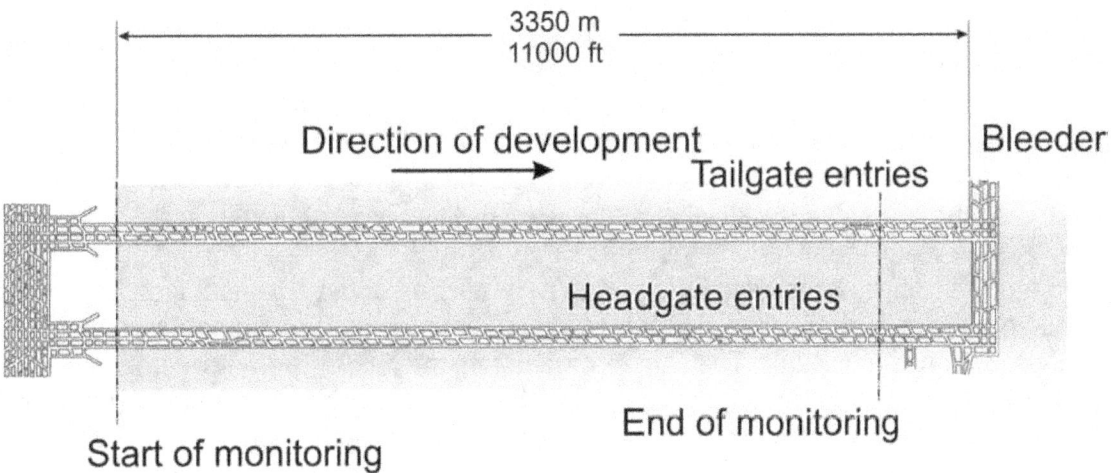

Figure 1.—The modeled longwall panel showing entry sections where mining and ventilation data were gathered during development mining.

Table 1.—Development mining parameters and their range of values used for modeling purposes

Mining parameter	Range of values
Mining height, ft	5.0–7.0
Entry development length, ft	1,000–12,000
Mining rate, ft/day	25–175
Methane concentration in mine air, %	0.5–1.5
Distance of shielding wells to entries, ft	19–87
Duration of degasification before mining, days	0–180

Table 2.—Coalbed reservoir properties and their range of values

Coalbed reservoir parameter	Base value	Range of values
Coalbed thickness, ft	6.0	5.0, 6.0, 7.0
Coalbed reservoir pressure, psi	90	90, 200, 400
Sorption time, days	20	20, 125, 250
Permeability anisotropy, K_x/K_y	4	4, 8
Face cleat permeability, K_x, md	4	4, 20, 40
Butt cleat permeability, K_y, md	1	0.5, 1.0, 2.5, 5.0, 10.0
Langmuir volume, scf/ton	392	200, 392, 600
Langmuir pressure, psi	326	126, 326, 526
Initial water saturation, S_{wi}, %	60	40, 60, 100
Effective porosity, %	4	0.5, 2, 4, 5
Irreducible water saturation, Sw_{ir}, %	40	10, 30, 40, 58
Relative permeability to gas (K_{rg}) at $S_g = 1 - Sw_{ir}$	0.35	0.35, 0.50, 0.70, 0.90

Effects of Mining Rate and Degasification Borehole Production on Methane Inflow

In-seam horizontal boreholes are effective in degasifying coal during development mining. To simulate the shielding effects of degasification wells on methane inflow and on the ventilation air requirements, 7.6-cm (3-in) diameter horizontal boreholes with no wellbore skin were modeled and operated with a negative bottom-hole pressure of 1,400 Pa (0.2 psi) for premining degasification periods of 0 months (i.e., no premining degasification), 3 months, and 6 months. Instead of the conventional distance used by industry, the boreholes were placed 5.8–27 m (19–90 ft) away from the entries to demonstrate the importance of proximity to effective emission reductions. In all cases, the boreholes were drilled ahead of development workings and operated as gate road entries were developed.

Figure 2 compares methane inflow rates as a function of development length for horizontal boreholes located 5.8 m (19 ft) away from the intake and return entries and operated for various premining durations. The data represent a 21-m/day (70-ft/day) development rate in a 2.1-m (7-ft) thick coalbed. Simulations show that the methane emissions into the development entries are highest when shielding degasification boreholes are not used before or during mining. Emission rates progressively decrease with increases in the duration of degasification. For instance, even if the boreholes did not operate before mining and begin to operate when mining starts, the inflow rate decreases about 25% compared to the completely unshielded case. The methane inflow rates to the ventilation air are lowest when longer premining degasification times are applied.

> **Emission rates in development entries decrease as a result of degasification. Even if the boreholes are placed just before mining, the methane rate in the ventilation air decreases about 25% compared to unshielded entries. However, larger emission decreases are possible.**

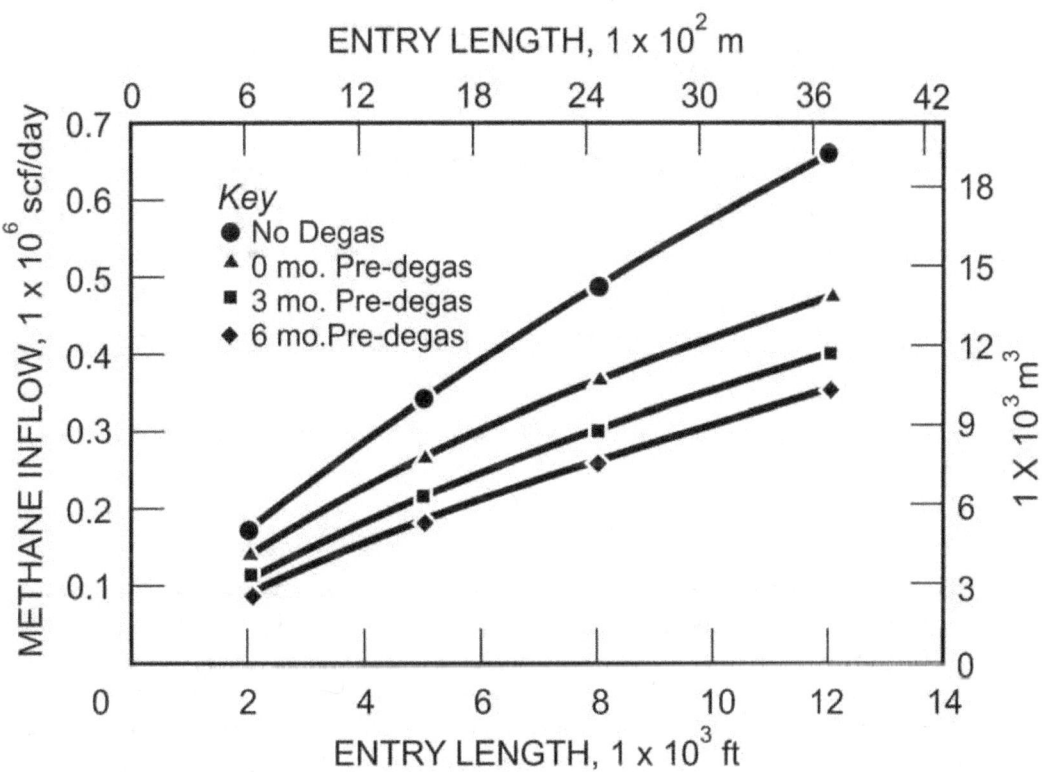

Figure 2.—Methane inflow rate predictions for different development lengths and various premining degasification durations.

The simulated data shown in Figure 3 are based on a 21-m/day (70-ft/day) development rate in a 2.1-m (7-ft) thick coalbed after 6 months of premining degasification, except for the "No wells present" case, which does not have any shielding. This figure shows that wellbores closest to the entries are most effective in reducing methane inflow rates during development mining, about 50% at 3,660 m (12,000 ft) compared to no shielding.

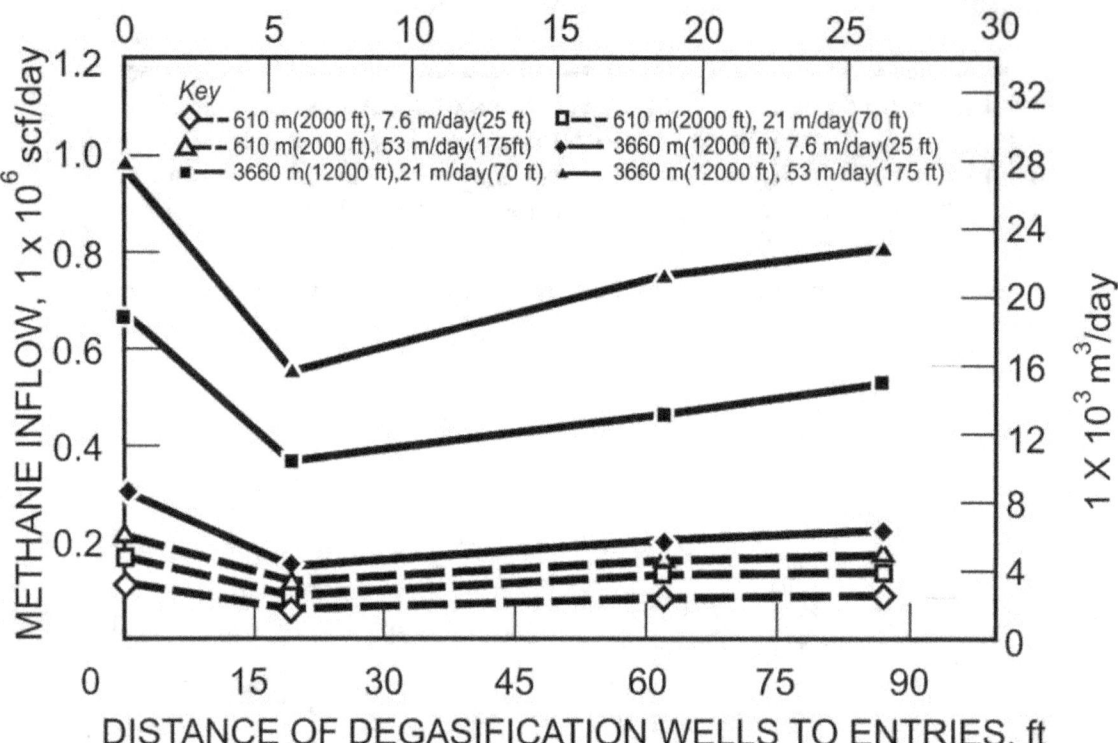

Figure 3.—Effect of mining rate and shielding well proximity when mining 610-m and 3,660-m (2,000-ft and 12,000-ft) long entries.

> **Shielding wells located close to gate road entries and operated for longer times are the most effective method in reducing the methane inflow rate into the development entries. Mine operators mining longer entries at higher mining rates will experience the greatest emissions reduction when applying this technology.**

Figure 3 also shows that the methane inflow rate increases with the length of the development section because of the increase in surface area of the exposed coalbed. This increase is strongly related to the mining rate. However, the effect of the mining rate on methane inflow is less pronounced for shorter development distances than for longer distances [Karacan et al. 2007a].

> The coalbed methane inflow rate increases with the length of the development section. The magnitude of the increase is strongly influenced by the mining rate, about 23,500 m³/day (1 × 10⁶ scf/day) with wells 25 m (82 ft) from the development heading. However, the effect of the mining rate on methane inflow is less pronounced for shorter development distances (610 m (2,000 ft)) than for longer entries.

Effects of Coalbed Parameters on Methane Inflow

The following subsections summarize the impacts of changing coalbed reservoir parameters (Table 2) on methane inflow. For these simulations, a 15-m/day (50-ft/day) section advance rate was assumed.

Coalbed Permeability and Permeability Anisotropy

Permeability is an intrinsic property of porous formations that relates pressure drop and flow rate. Coalbeds are characterized as anisotropic reservoirs with two orthogonal permeability components that run in the direction of characteristic fractures within the coalbed. These are termed the "face cleats" and "butt cleats." Face cleats are continuous and can extend for long distances. Butt cleats are short and discontinuous, usually terminating at face cleats. Due to the nature of these two cleat systems, face cleats are more permeable to gas and water flow. Vertical permeability is usually significantly lower than horizontal permeability. Thus, horizontal permeability and its direction are more important in coalbed reservoirs. The permeability anisotropy can be defined as the ratio of face cleat to butt cleat permeabilities. The presence, lack, or direction of permeability has a profound effect on methane inflow into the wellbores [Remner et al. 1986], suggesting that any horizontal drilling in coalbeds should account for directional permeability. The average permeability for flow in coalbeds can be defined as

$$K_a = \sqrt{K_x \times K_y} \tag{1}$$

where K_a is the average permeability, and K_x and K_y are the directional permeabilities of the cleats.

Direction and magnitude of permeability are important for control of methane emissions during mining. When mining advances perpendicular to the face cleats, where permeability is higher, much more gas is emitted into mine workings than when the advance is parallel to the face cleat. In fact, in one area of a mine operating in the Pittsburgh coalbed, the methane emission from the solid ribs was significantly higher than that from the working face as a result of the ribs intersecting the face cleats [McCulloch et al. 1975].

11

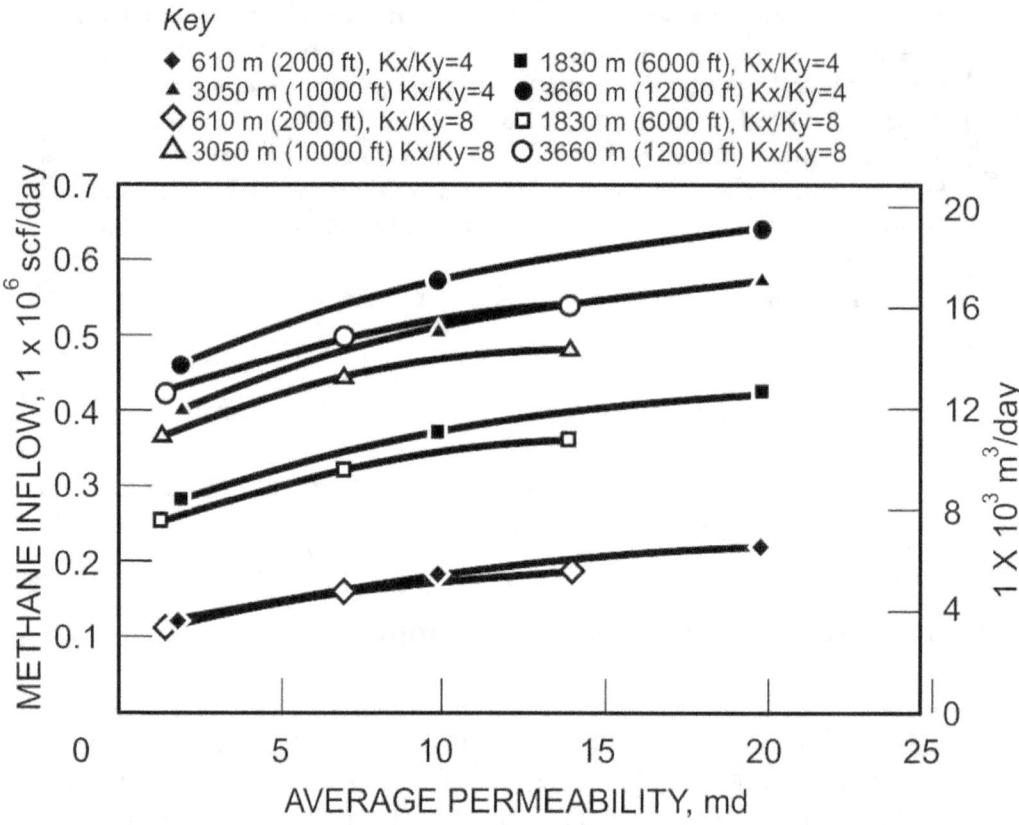

Figure 4.—Reservoir model predictions of methane inflow rate changes with permeability, permeability anisotropy, and entry length.

Figure 4 shows that increasing average permeability, while keeping the anisotropy constant, increases methane inflow into the entries. On the other hand, when anisotropy is doubled, methane inflow decreases, even though the face cleat permeability remains the same. This is due to a lower flow rate from the decreased butt cleat permeability where the butt cleat is perpendicular to the entries in this study. Also, Figure 4 shows that the effects of anisotropy or changes in butt cleat permeability are more pronounced for longer development distances. In a more general sense, the effect of butt cleat permeability observed in this study should be interpreted as the effect of coalbed permeability in the cleat system, which is perpendicular to the entries based on orientation of mining.

> The permeability of cleats perpendicular to the mine entries is more important in controlling methane inflow rates than the maximum face cleat permeability.

Langmuir Volume, Langmuir Pressure, and Coalbed Pressure

In coalbeds, the major portion of the gas exists in the adsorbed state within the coal matrix rather than in a free state within the cleats. As the pressure is lowered due to fluid production from the cleats, gas starts to desorb from the micropore surfaces and diffuse into the macropores [Remner et al. 1986]. Adsorption and desorption of methane from coal is described by a Langmuir isotherm that defines the relationship of coalbed pressure to the capacity of a given coal to hold gas at a constant temperature. More specifically, the Langmuir isotherm for coals relates matrix gas content, $V(P)$, to the coalbed cleat pressure, P, according to:

$$V(P) = \frac{V_L \times P}{(P + P_L)} \tag{2}$$

V_L is the Langmuir volume or maximum amount of gas that can be adsorbed. Langmuir pressure, P_L, is a measurement strongly related to the residence time for a gas molecule on a coal surface and represents the pressure at which gas storage capacity is half of the maximum storage capacity, V_L [Young 1998]. Both V_L and P_L can be determined from gas sorption measurements on the coal core samples. The Langmuir equation (Equation 2) provides a necessary boundary condition at the matrix-cleat interface [Young 1998]. For nonequilibrium diffusion sorption models, it is assumed that the concentration of methane at the surface of the micropore matrix blocks is in equilibrium with the free gas pressure in the cleats. This implies that the external boundary condition of the micropore equation is the equilibrium sorption isotherm [King et al. 1986]. The shape of this isotherm is important for manipulating the boundary condition between matrix and cleats and for controlling the desorption rate of gas from coal.

> **Coalbed methane emission rates are strongly influenced by methane content. The gas content of a coal at a range of coalbed pressures is controlled by the Langmuir isotherm, relating Langmuir volume, V_L, and Langmuir pressure, P_L. Cleat pressure is also important for determining the gas content of the coalbed for a given V_L and P_L.**

It should be noted that initially the actual amount of gas in the coalbed (gas content) may not be on the desorption curve defined by the Langmuir isotherm, but may be below this curve. In this case, coalbed cleat pressure needs to be reduced further until it reaches a critical desorption pressure where gas starts to desorb and gas release follows the Langmuir isotherm as pressure declines.

To obtain the data in Figure 5, mining advance was oriented parallel to the face cleats to mimic the modeled mine. Both face and butt cleat permeabilities were varied between the minimum and maximum values shown in Table 2. Permeability anisotropies were increased by decreasing the butt cleat permeability.

Figure 5 shows the effect of coalbed pressure on the methane inflow rate during the development mining of gate road entries. A higher coalbed gas or hydrostatic pressure results in a higher methane inflow rate at constant V_L and P_L. The dependency of inflow rate on pressure is nearly linear for each of the entry lengths studied. Also, the inflow rate is higher when mining longer entries, as expected, since longer entries create a larger drainage area into which gas can flow. Furthermore, a much larger portion of the coal seam is depressurized sooner, which triggers gas desorption from greater distances. A similar phenomenon is observed when increasing the length of horizontal coalbed production wells [Ertekin et al. 1988; King et al. 1986].

The effects of V_L and P_L on simulated methane inflow into the entries during development mining are shown in Figure 6. This figure shows that methane inflow rate is almost a linear function of V_L. Since V_L represents the maximum gas capacity of coal, higher V_L ensures the availability of more methane and promotes higher methane emissions when pressure and P_L are kept constant. The variable P_L shows an inverse relationship with the methane inflow rate when both V_L and pressure are constant (Figure 6). The slope of the isotherm, or the change of gas capacity with pressure, is largely controlled by P_L. As P_L increases, then the isotherm will be flat compared to an isotherm generated from a coal sample with a lower P_L value. This means that when mining a coalbed with a higher P_L, the change in gas capacity or change in gas desorption from the coal will be less compared to a seam with a lower P_L for the same pressure drop. Thus, the rates of desorption and methane inflow into entries in a higher-P_L coalbed decrease as development distances increase.

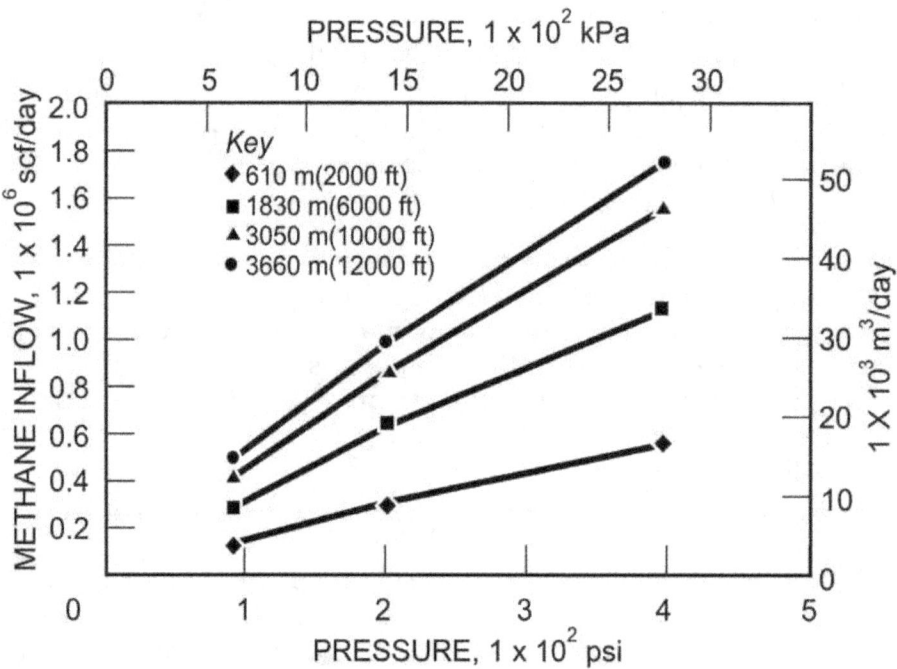

Figure 5.—Effects of coalbed pressure on predicted methane inflow rates into development entries using reservoir simulations.

14

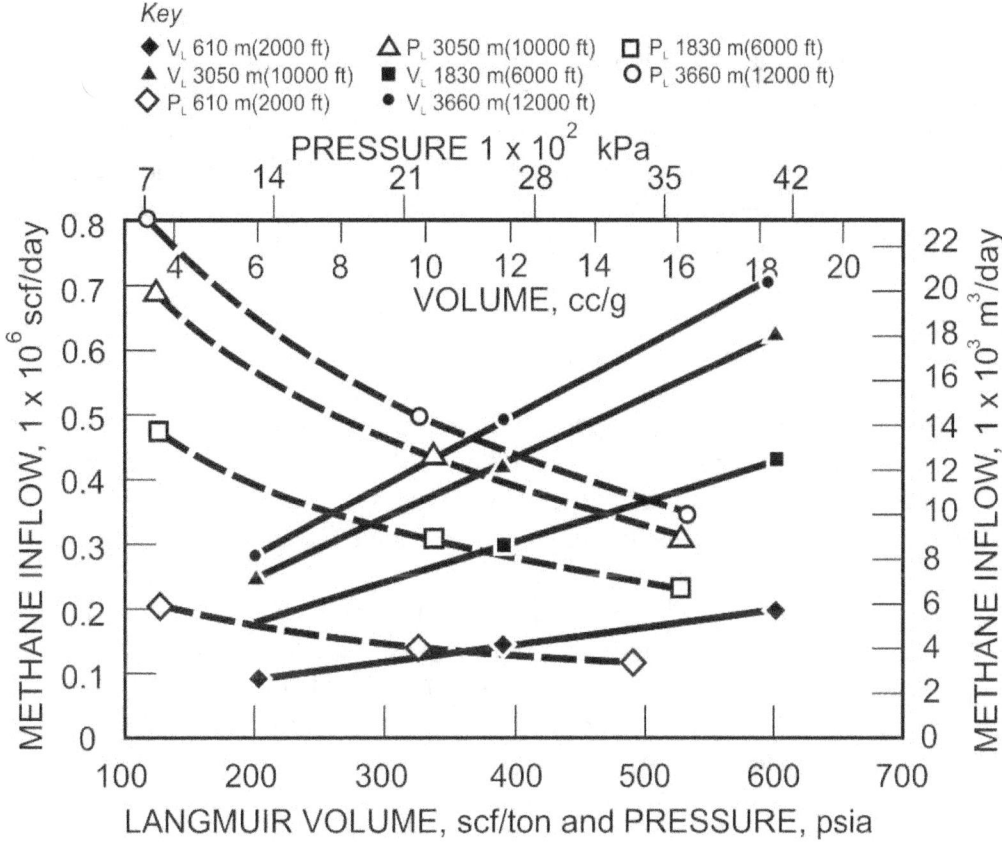

Figure 6.—Effects of Langmuir pressure (P_L) and Langmuir volume (V_L) on simulated methane inflow rates.

> **Methane emission rates are an almost linear function of pressure and the distance to be mined. Simulations show that a higher Langmuir volume V_L ensures the availability of more methane and promotes a higher methane drainage rate when pressure and Langmuir pressure, P_L, are kept constant. The inverse is true with a higher Langmuir pressure.**

Sorption Time Constant

Once methane desorbs from the micropore surfaces of a coal matrix, it flows through the micropores in response to a methane concentration gradient defined by a combination of Knudsen, bulk, and surface diffusion processes [Smith and Williams 1984; Kolesar and Ertekin 1986]. In coalbed modeling, unsteady-state diffusion effects can be quantified by determining a sorption time, τ (days), which is related to cleat spacing, s_f, and the diffusion coefficient, D:

$$\tau \sim \frac{s_f^2}{D} \tag{3}$$

15

In effect, τ is the time constant that regulates the rate at which gas is released from the micropores into the macropore system. For small values of τ, or larger values of D, the diffusion and sorption process is faster, and a higher cumulative gas production and a higher production rate peak are observed at degasification boreholes [Remner et al. 1986; Spencer et al. 1987]. Later in the life of the coalbed methane reservoir, sorption time, together with desorption, may also act as an internal pressure maintenance mechanism.

The simulated effects of different sorption times are shown in Figure 7, which demonstrate that small sorption times cause higher methane inflow rates, as observed in gas production from coalbeds using horizontal boreholes [Remner et al. 1986]. It is also evident that the change in inflow rates between short and long sorption times is more significant as entry lengths increase. This relationship may be related to the regulation of the rate of gas release from micropores to cleats and the gas pressure distribution in the reservoir during active mining. When the entries being mined are relatively short, the pressure disturbance within the coalbed is more limited and the area of methane drainage is diminished. When mining longer entries, the inflow rates are higher because the pressure disturbance affects a larger area for a longer time and a larger surface area is exposed. A short sorption time, τ, results in high gas flow rates from the areas surrounding the entries and from the areas where pressure transients can propagate. In the case of longer sorption times, the flow rate will be less due to slow diffusion from the coal matrices into the cleats. Also, the pressure transients will travel farther since there will not be enough pressure maintenance in the coalbed.

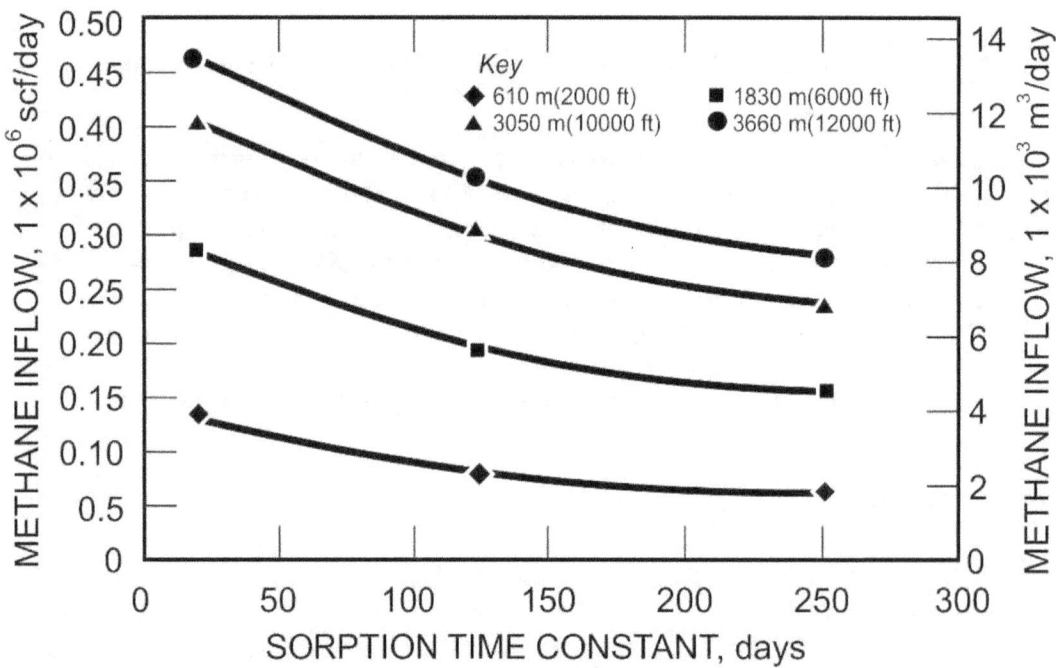

Figure 7.—Influence of sorption time constant of the coal on reservoir-simulated methane inflow rates during mining.

> **Small sorption times cause higher methane inflow rates into gate road entries. The effect of the sorption time constant on methane inflow rates into mine workings is more significant for the mining of longer entries than for shorter ones.**

Coalbed Thickness

Figure 8 shows that the methane inflow rates increase almost linearly with the coalbed thickness. The figure also shows that, as expected, mining longer entries in thicker coalbeds results in higher inflow rates. This is due to a combination of the two factors suggested by Ertekin et al. [1988] for fracture-stimulated horizontal boreholes: the reservoir volume is larger and the surface area for gas flow is increased in fracture-stimulated horizontal boreholes. Ertekin et al. reported that methane production from horizontal boreholes increases as the coalbed thickness increases even if the borehole surface area is the same because of larger volumes of reserves encountered.

During development mining in thicker coalbeds, larger volumes of methane reserves are encountered. Also, the increased thickness of the coalbed results in an increased area of flow due to the presence of the natural fracture network. Thus, when mining longer entries, increased magnitudes of reserves that are encountered and larger surface areas created combine for increasing inflow rates even further.

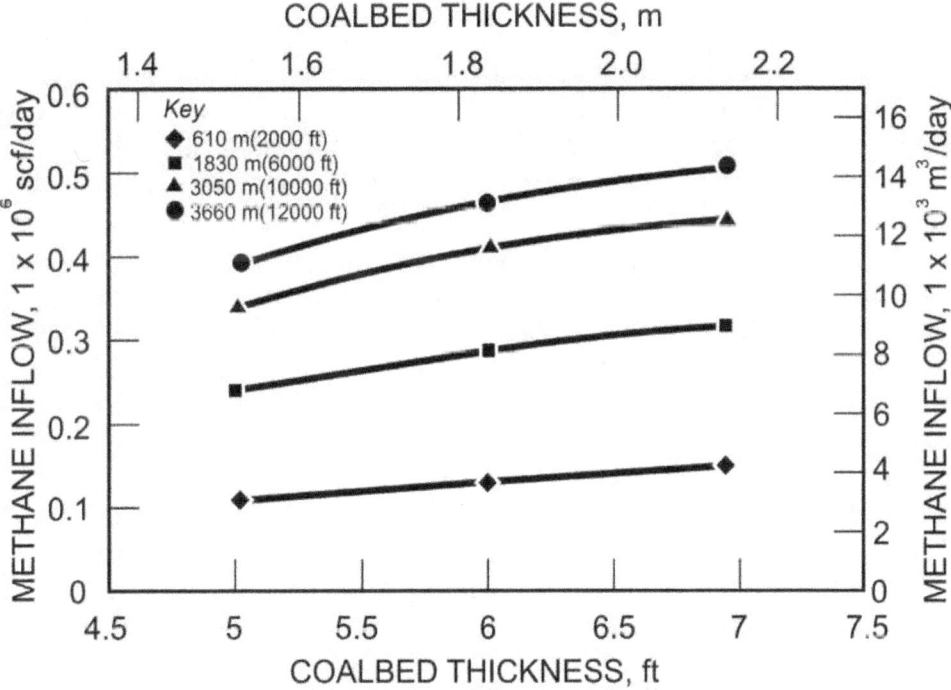

Figure 8.—Effect of coalbed thickness on predicted methane inflow rates into entries of various lengths using reservoir simulation models.

Initial Water Saturation of the Coalbed

Coalbeds are almost always partially or completely saturated with water. However, since porosity and permeability of coal matrices are extremely low, almost all of the water resides in fractures and cleats in the coalbed. Thus, any water saturation for coalbeds represents the fraction of cleat porosity that is occupied by water. The definition of saturation is based on the total pore volume of cleats. A fraction of the pore volume may be occupied by immobile water, where water saturation cannot be reduced further. Thus, water saturation in cleats may vary between a minimum value (immobile water saturation) and a maximum of 100% saturation.

Simulation work by Karacan [forthcoming] showed that reducing irreducible water saturation to 10% for a development distance of 610 m (2,000 ft) reduced the methane inflow rate. Increasing initial water saturation, while keeping other parameters constant at their base values, had a more significant effect on methane inflow rates. When mining 610- and 1,830-m (2,000- and 6,000-ft) entries, increasing initial water saturation decreased methane inflow rate due to decreased initial gas saturations and gas relative permeabilities. A similar decrease was observed in the longer entries when initial water saturation was changed from 40% to 80%.

> **It is critical to the successful reduction of underground emission rates to remove water from a coalbed in the process of producing coalbed methane from a borehole. The initial water saturation of a coalbed has a more significant effect on methane inflow rates in the mining of shorter entries (about 1,830 m (6,000 ft) or less).**

When mining 3,050-m and 3,660-m (10,000-ft and 12,000-ft) long gate roads, gas inflow rate increased when water saturation was increased from 80% to 100%. This may be related to capturing negative decline and the peak rates of methane from the coalbed during the dewatering phase. When the coalbed is partially saturated with water, both water and methane are produced concurrently, and inflow of methane from cleats into the entries may show a declining trend with time. When mining begins in a coalbed that is 100% saturated with water, water will initially flow into the entries rapidly and trigger a high gas inflow rate as in the "negative decline" period of production wells, thus increasing average inflow rate into the entries. Shorter entry developments may not experience the effect of this period, and inflow rate may decrease due to water saturation. However, mining longer entries gives sufficient time and longer coalbed exposure for the high gas inflow rate experienced during negative decline to impact average methane inflow [Karacan, forthcoming].

Karacan [forthcoming] used multiple regression to assess the relationships between methane inflow rates and various coalbed reservoir parameters (Table 3). Methane inflow rates were calculated for 610-to 3,660-m (2,000- to 12,000-ft) gate road lengths assuming a 15-m/day (50-ft/day) section advance rate. The units of coalbed parameters are presented in Table 1. These analyses revealed that sorption time constant, butt-cleat permeability, and Langmuir pressure were found to be the most influential on methane inflow rates for all gate road lengths. For shorter gate road lengths, initial water saturation was also found to impact methane inflow rates [Karacan, forthcoming].

Table 3.—Linear models for predicting methane inflow rates into development entries of various lengths using key coalbed reservoir parameters

Entry length (ft)	Methane inflow rate (scf/day) =	R^2
2,000	$-9025.0349 + (18676.8392 \times$ Thick) $+ (1367.1790 \times$ Pres) $+ (-581.1950 \times$ S.Time) $+ (13100.6770 \times K_y) +$ $(121.6918 \times$ L.Vol.) $+ (-197.1251 \times$ L.Pres.) $+$ $(-1280.3404 \times$ W.Sat.)	0.9209
6,000	$-193021.37 + (49697.1335 \times$ Thick) $+ (2734.4987 \times$ Pres) $+ (-997.3667 \times$ S.Time) $+ (19103.2963 \times K_y) +$ $(298.3296 \times$ L.Vol.) $+ (-544.3628 \times$ L.Pres.)	0.9011
10,000	$-256242.06 + (73838.2649 \times$ Thick) $+ (3764.7566 \times$ Pres) $+ (-1256.0067 \times$ S.Time) $+ (21052.8924 \times K_y) +$ $(457.1441 \times$ L.Vol.) $+ (-867.7456 \times$ L.Pres.)	0.8896
12,000	$-283185.59 + (85055.0763 \times$ Thick) $+ (4219.7519 \times$ Pres) $+ (-1357.3077 \times$ S.Time) $+ (21403.8583 \times K_y) +$ $(532.4142 \times$ L.Vol.) $+ (-1023.3603 \times$ L.Pres.)	0.8844

Thick = Thickness; Pres = Pressure; S.Time = Sorption time constant; K_y = Butt cleat permeability in this study, but can be interpreted as the cleat permeability perpendicular to entries; L.Vol. = Langmuir volume; L.Pres. = Langmuir pressure; W.Sat. = Water saturation.

NOTE.—Regression was performed using U.S. customary units of measure.

Summary

- The coalbed methane inflow rate increases with the length of the development section and is strongly influenced by the mining rate.

- Shielding degasification boreholes decrease the methane inflow rate in the ventilation air compared to unshielded entries, even if operational only during the mining cycle.

- Shielding wells located close to gate road entries and operated for longer times are the most effective method application of this methane drainage technology.

- Coalbed methane emission rates are strongly influenced by methane content. The gas content of a coal at a range of coalbed pressures is controlled by the Langmuir isotherm.

- Methane emission rates are an almost linear function of pressure and the distance to be mined.

- The permeability of cleats perpendicular to the mine entries is more important in controlling methane inflow rates than the maximum face cleat permeability.

- The effect of the sorption time constant on methane inflow rates into mine workings is more significant for longer entries than for shorter ones.

19

- The initial water saturation of a coalbed has a more significant effect on methane inflow rates in the mining of shorter entries.

- The coalbed parameters that most strongly influence methane emission rates for short entries under 610 m (2,000 ft) are, in decreasing importance:

  1. Reservoir pressure
  2. Sorption time constant
  3. Permeability
  4. Langmuir pressure
  5. Langmuir volume
  6. Thickness
  7. Water saturation

- For long entries (3,660 m (12,000 ft)), the most important parameters are:

  1. Reservoir pressure
  2. Sorption time constant
  3. Langmuir pressure
  4. Thickness
  5. Permeability
  6. Langmuir volume

2. CONTROLLING LONGWALL FACE METHANE AND DEVELOPMENT MINING EMISSIONS: PREDICTED IMPROVEMENTS USING IN-SEAM BOREHOLES

Overview

This section focuses on the optimization of methane drainage technology aimed at reducing and controlling longwall face emission rates and concentrations. Reservoir modeling software has been used to assess methane drainage methods, which are all based on the application of in-seam boreholes that are rotary or directionally drilled. The boreholes are drilled ahead of mining, and coalbed methane production is terminated prior to being mined through by the longwall face. The modeling results provide a comparison for the production and emissions reductions that can be expected from different borehole configurations over a range of gas production durations.

As mines progress into deeper and gassier coalbeds, or as longwall panel size increases, ventilation and GGVs together may not be sufficient to maintain methane levels within statutory limits. To decrease the explosion risk associated with methane emissions under these circumstances, in-seam horizontal methane drainage is often used to reduce the gas content of the coalbed prior to mining. Degasification of the coalbed prior to mining is effective in reducing face emission rates and volumes (emissions from the freshly exposed face of the coalbed, broken coal pieces during mining, and the coal load on the conveyor belts). Potentially, if enough time elapses after gate road development and prior to longwall mining, gas emissions into the development entries from the panel may help reduce future gas emissions during panel extraction [Diamond and Garcia 1999]. However, there may not always be enough time for the coalbed to drain before the longwall starts production. This is especially true since longwall productivity has increased considerably in recent years because of advances in mining methods and machinery. Aul and Ray [1991] reported that longwall productivity increased by 200%–400% between 1983 and 1990; the accompanying methane emissions increased by as much as 200%–300% in several mines operating at depths ranging from 370 to 730 m (1,200 to 2,400 ft) in the Pocahontas No. 3 Coalbed in Virginia.

To investigate these issues, a reservoir model was developed and calibrated for a longwall mining area in the Pittsburgh Coalbed in Greene County, PA. The study area at the mine was located in a new mining district where panels were initially 381 m (1,250 ft) wide and were increased to 442 m (1,450 ft) starting with the third panel. The study site is described in greater detail by Karacan et al. [2007a].

A methane drainage program using in-seam horizontal boreholes in the Pittsburgh Coalbed is used at the study site to shield the gate roads during development and to reduce the in-place methane content of the outlined longwall panel. As the gate roads advance, two to three sets of two horizontal boreholes are generally drilled from what will eventually be the tailgate entries of each panel. The number of sets depends generally on the length of the panels and the length of the individual boreholes. The holes are drilled toward what will be the startup end of each panel, with one hole paralleling the tailgate side of the panel. The individual horizontal boreholes are connected to a common underground pipeline for transmission to the surface [Karacan et al. 2007a].

Five different horizontal, in-seam, methane drainage borehole patterns were evaluated in this study (Figure 9, A through E). The gate road entries shown represent a three-entry system with intervening coal pillars. The boreholes in patterns C and D were spaced equally. In all of the patterns, each borehole was modeled as a 7.6-cm (3-in) diameter, unstimulated well drilled from the tailgate entries into the Pittsburgh Coalbed. The total lengths of the simulated boreholes were 5,610 m, 8,480 m, 1,160 m, 2,320 m, and 1,840 m (18,400 ft, 27,800 ft, 3,800 ft, 7,600 ft, and 6,050 ft) for patterns A, B, C, D, and E, respectively. The boreholes operated at bottom-hole pressures equal to atmospheric pressure to represent the absence of any exhausters used to aid gas flow. To evaluate gas production potential during mining, the 3- and 12-month premining methane drainage models for each borehole pattern were extended by 268 days to include the production of gas during extraction of the longwall panel [Karacan et al. 2007a].

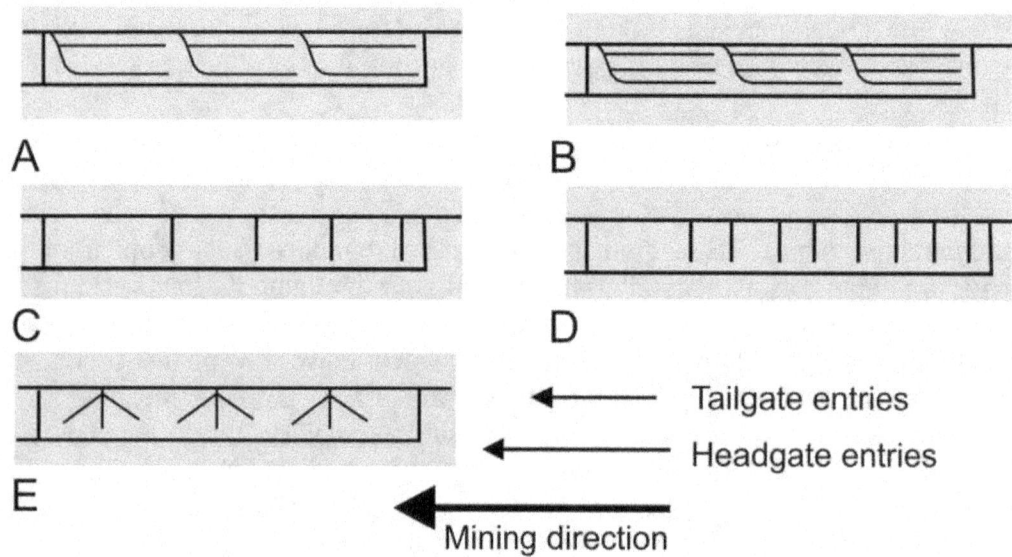

Figure 9.—Horizontal methane drainage borehole patterns modeled for degasification of the longwall panel *(not to scale)*.

The horizontal borehole production data were evaluated to estimate the potential average reductions in face emission rates as a result of premining methane drainage. The calculated average face emission reductions were also determined. For this calculation, cumulative methane production was divided by the duration (268 days) of mining for the study panel. The assumption was that either the majority (75%) or the total (100%) of the methane produced would be released as face emissions during mining if it was not removed prior to mining. This assumption is based on the work of Noack [1998], who proposed that, in the absence of empirical data, the degree of gas emission (percentage of gas-in-place) could be assumed to be 100% in stratigraphic zones within 20 to −11 m (66 to −36 ft) of the top and bottom of the mined coalbed, and 75% in the mined coalbed. The calculated average face emission rates that can be expected if methane drainage is not utilized are 27 m³/min (940 cfm) for the 100% gas emission basis and 20 m³/min (710 cfm) for the 75% emission basis. These predictions are based on the calculated total in-place methane content of 10×10^6 m³ (360 MMscf) in the outlined panel and 268 days of longwall mining.

Using horizontal borehole pattern B in the Pittsburgh Coalbed reduces the average face emission rates by as much as 10 m³/min (360 cfm) for the 100% emission basis and by

7.6 m^3/min (270 cfm) for the 75% basis after 12 months of premining degasification. The methane emission reduction values for pattern A are as much as 6.8 m^3/min (240 cfm) for the 100% basis and 5.1 m^3/min (180 cfm) for the 75% basis. The possible face emission reduction values calculated for D are 6.2 and 4.5 m^3/min (220 and 160 cfm) for the 100% and 75% basis respectively, after 12 months of degasification. Lesser amounts of face emission reductions are calculated for patterns C and E. Figure 10 compares cumulative methane productions, different horizontal borehole patterns, and the reductions in face emission rates for the 100% degree of gas emission basis.

The overall reduction in average face emission rates due to methane drainage can be evaluated by analyzing the panel extraction phase and combining it with premining methane drainage performance. After 12 months of premining degasification, the additional reductions in face emissions with continued degasification during mining are 0.9 m^3/min and 1.2 m^3/min (32 and 42 cfm) for the 100% basis with patterns A and B, respectively. The additional face emission reduction that can be achieved with patterns D and E due to continued degasification is similar to that of A (0.8 and 0.7 m^3/min (28 and 25 cfm), respectively), and the reduction is less with C after 12 months of premining degasification.

The data in Table 4 show that after only 3 months of premining degasification, continued degasification during panel extraction becomes more important. For instance, after 3 months of premining degasification, continued methane drainage during mining using borehole pattern A reduces face emission rates by 1.8 m^3/min (64 cfm) for the 100% degree of emission basis and 1.4 m^3/min (49 cfm) for the 75% basis. These reductions are more than 50% of what can be achieved in addition to 3 months of premining degasification. Similar impacts are achieved with other borehole patterns as well as a result of continued degasification during panel extraction after a short (3-month) premining degasification period.

After 3 months of premining degasification, additional drainage during mining using borehole pattern B reduces face emission rates by 2.7 m^3/min (95 cfm) for the 100% emission basis and 2.1 m^3/min (74 cfm) for the 75% basis. These data (Table 4) show that additional degasification after a 3-month premining production period with pattern B is almost as effective as pattern A.

Table 4.—Simulated reductions in face emission rates after different phases of methane drainage using horizontal boreholes from the longwall panel

	Pre-mining degasifi-cation, months	Wellbore pattern[1]									
		A		B		C		D		E	
		100% emis-sion, cfm	75% emis-sion, cfm	100% emis-sion, cfm	75% emis-sion, cfm	100% emis-sion, cfm	75% emis-sion, cfm	100% emis-sion, cfm	75% emis-sion, cfm	100% emis-sion, cfm	75% emis-sion, cfm
Premining degasification	3	100	78	160	120	49	35	92	67	71	53
	12	240	180	360	270	110	85	220	160	180	130
Degasification during mining	3	64	49	95	74	25	18	57	42	49	35
	12	32	21	42	32	14	11	28	21	25	18
Total emissions reduction	3	164	130	255	190	74	53	149	110	120	92
	12	272	200	402	310	124	95	248	180	205	150

[1]From Figure 9.

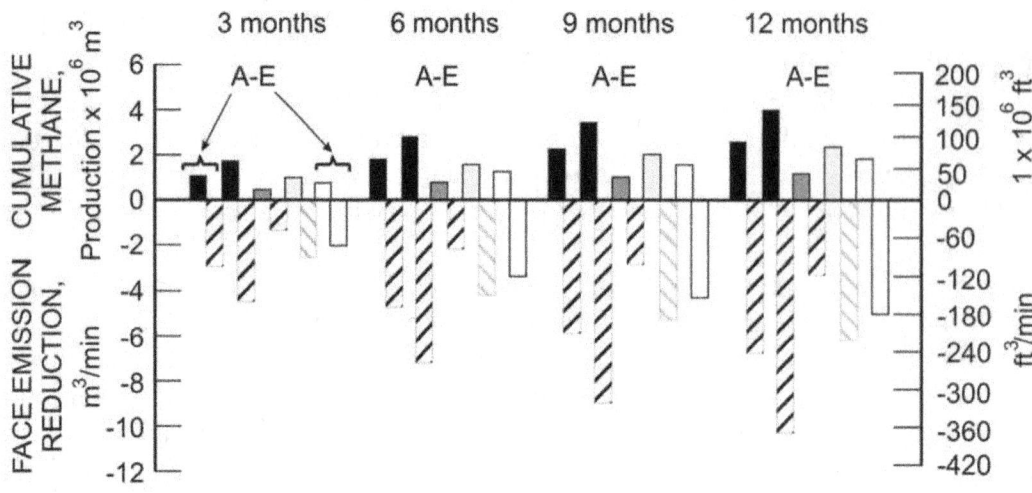

Figure 10.—Cumulative methane production and possible reductions in longwall face emission rates for different premining methane drainage time intervals and different horizontal borehole patterns (A through E).

The total reductions in average face emissions after 12 months of methane drainage before and during mining are significant, particularly with horizontal borehole patterns A, B, and D. The total reduction that can be achieved with pattern B is between 8.8 and 12 m^3/min (310 and 410 cfm). This reduction can decrease the average maximum emission rate that may be expected from the Pittsburgh Coalbed from 20–27 m^3/min (710–940 cfm) to less than 11–15 m^3/min (400–540 cfm).

> **Longer degasification times result in lower face emission rates. For the Pittsburgh Coalbed, the most effective borehole pattern is the trilateral configuration (pattern B), followed by the dual-lateral arrangement (pattern A). High emission reductions can also be achieved or exceeded by a large number of short, cross-panel boreholes drilled in a closely spaced, linear manner.**

During simulation of longwall degasification, GGVs were put into production as the longwall face advanced to their location [Karacan et al. 2007a]. Figure 11 shows methane production from the simulated horizontal methane drainage borehole patterns shown in Figure 9 before and during panel extraction. The results show that methane production during panel extraction is substantially less than that of the premining phase. Additionally, as the premining degasification time increases from 3 to 12 months, the amount of methane produced by the horizontal boreholes during panel extraction decreases even more. The reduced methane production is probably due to a combination of two factors. First, the methane content of the coalbed is reduced during the premining methane drainage phase, leaving less methane available for production at a slower rate during mining, especially after a longer premining degasification. Second, the methane production from each horizontal borehole is progressively terminated as the longwall face reaches its location [Karacan et al. 2007a]. The simulation results shown in

Figure 11 indicate that the highest cumulative methane production is achieved with long horizontal borehole patterns A and B. However, as the number of shorter, cross-panel, horizontal boreholes perpendicular to the higher-permeability face cleats increases, as in pattern D, their cumulative production approaches that of pattern A.

> **The period of premining degasification should be extended for as long as possible. Methane production during panel extraction is substantially less than that of the premining phase due to the decreased methane content of the coalbed and the successive termination of the boreholes during mining.**

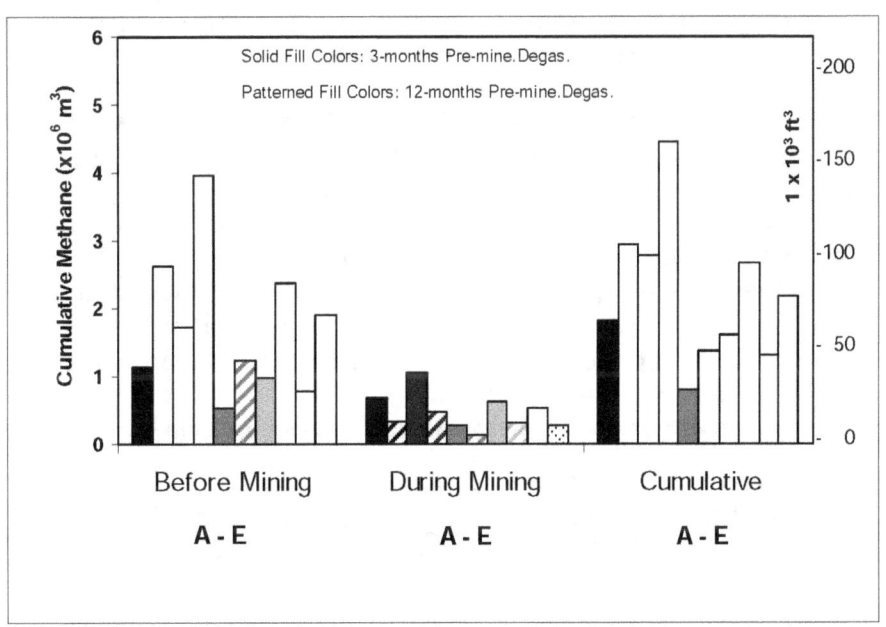

Figure 11.—Performances of different horizontal methane drainage borehole patterns shown in Figure 9 during different phases of degasification, after 3 and 12 months of premining degasification.

Effects of Methane Drainage on Longwall Face Emissions

The overall reduction in average face emission rates due to methane drainage can be evaluated by analyzing the panel extraction phase and combining it with premining methane drainage performance. The average reductions in longwall face emission rates due to methane drainage before and during mining were calculated and are shown in Figure 11 and Table 4. The data show that longwall face emissions were reduced by 11 m³/min (400 cfm) with 12 months of premining methane drainage using borehole pattern B. As would be expected, the simulations show that 3 months of premining methane drainage is less effective in reducing the total emission rate than 12 months of premining drainage.

After 12 months of premining degasification, the additional reductions in face emissions with continued degasification during mining are 0.9 m^3/min and 1.2 m^3/min (32 and 42 cfm) for the 100% basis with patterns A and B, respectively. The data in Table 4 show that after only 3 months of premining degasification, continued degasification during panel extraction becomes more important.

The data presented in Table 4 show that after 3 months of premining degasification, continued methane drainage during mining using borehole pattern A reduces face emission rates by 1.8 m^3/min (64 cfm) for the 100% degree of emission basis and 1.4 m^3/min (49 cfm) for the 75% basis. These reductions are more than 50% of what can be achieved in addition to 3 months of premining degasification. Similar impacts are achieved with other borehole patterns as well as a result of continued degasification during panel extraction after a short (3-month) premining degasification period. On the other hand, the incremental reduction obtained with continued degasification during panel extraction in average face emission rates after 12 months of pre-mining degasification using the same borehole pattern is about 15% of what can be achieved by 12 months premining degasification. Again, similar reductions in average face emissions were observed for the other borehole patterns after continued degasification.

> **It is important to continue methane drainage during mining to maximize reductions in longwall face methane emissions. Methane borehole production during panel extraction and its resultant effect on face emissions is substantially less than during the premining phase. However, if the duration of pre-mining methane drainage is short, the contribution of methane produced during panel extraction and the subsequent face emission reduction may be significant.**

Effectiveness of Shielding the Development Entries From Methane Migration and Emissions

In-seam methane drainage boreholes not only degas the longwall panel itself, but can also shield the advancing development entries from methane emissions from the surrounding virgin coalbed gas reservoir [Diamond 1994]. To study this phenomenon, the impacts of borehole pattern on the effectiveness of shielding gate roads from methane migration were evaluated. In this analysis, two approaches were used. In the first approach, methane emissions were predicted in conjunction with operating in-seam horizontal methane drainage boreholes, configured as shown in Figure 9. In the second approach, three horizontal boreholes were placed in the virgin coalbed along the gate roads on both sides of the outlined panel, as shown in Figure 12, for pattern A+ (applicable only to the first longwall panel in a new mining district) [Karacan et al. 2007a]. The first approach is intended to analyze the amount of methane migrating into the gate roads from the panel area and the surrounding coalbed only in the presence of in-panel horizontal methane drainage boreholes. The second approach analyzes the effects of additional boreholes on shielding the entries from methane emissions from the surrounding coalbed during premining degasification.

Table 5 gives the predicted methane inflow into the ventilation system from the surrounding virgin coalbed at the end of various methane drainage time intervals based on the presence of in-panel horizontal methane drainage boreholes (A+ to E+), along with methane inflow into the ventilation in the absence of any degasification borehole. These comparative results show that borehole patterns A and B, where near-margin horizontal boreholes are drilled from the tailgate, are more effective against methane inflow into the gate roads during premining degasification than the other patterns because of their extended length along the entries. The simulation indicates that by using either pattern A+ or B+, the potential methane inflow into the entries can be reduced by as much as $62 \times 10^4 \text{ m}^3$ $(22 \times 10^6 \text{ ft}^3)$ over 12 months, which corresponds to a decrease in methane inflow by ~1.1 m^3/min (~40 cfm) simply by shielding against methane inflow originating from the coalbed within the panel area. As would be expected, this suggests that the middle horizontal borehole segments in pattern B+ do not contribute much to gate road shielding.

The results of a borehole drilling study for shielding the entries from methane inflow were reported by DuBois et al. [2006]. This research was conducted in the Pittsburgh Coalbed at the same mining district modeled in this study. The horizontal boreholes of pattern A were drilled to maximize the shielding for both belt and return entries during headgate and tailgate development. This approach resulted in a pattern similar to the one designated as A+ in this study. The drilling strategy described by DuBois et al. permitted horizontal boreholes to be active for 6–24 months prior to any mining. They reported that methane concentration decreased by 41%, and methane emission into the entries decreased between 30% and 35%, close to the predicted values in this study for patterns A+ and B+.

> **The emissions into the gate road entries originate mostly from the gas desorbing from the margins of the panel where the in-seam, near-margin borehole segments are located and where these boreholes are most effective in capturing this gas.**

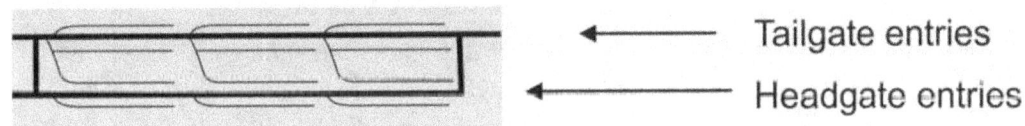

Figure 12.—Sample layout showing additional horizontal, in-seam boreholes on either side of the gate roads (A+) in addition to pattern A *(not to scale)*.

> **Additional reductions in methane emissions into the gate roads can be achieved by employing horizontal methane drainage boreholes in the surrounding virgin coalbed gas reservoir on either side of the gate roads. Methane migration into the mine ventilation airflow in the gate road entries surrounding the outlined longwall panel can be reduced effectively by using dual and trilateral horizontal methane drainage holes paralleling the gate roads.**

Table 5.—Predicted methane emissions into the ventilation system from the surrounding coalbed (within the panel and virgin coal)

Wellbore pattern	Methane inflow into mine ventilation system ($\times 10^6$ ft^3) for various durations of methane drainage			
	3 months	6 months	9 months	12 months
No degasification	78.8	126	159	186
A (A+)	74.5 (66.7)	116 (99.6)	144 (119)	164 (132)
B (B+)	74.5 (66.7)	116 (99.6)	144 (119)	164 (132)
C (C+)	78.0 (72.0)	124 (108)	156 (132)	181 (150)
D (D+)	77.3 (69.6)	123 (107)	155 (131)	179 (147)
E (E+)	78.0 (70.3)	124 (107)	156 (131)	178 (147)

NOTE.—"+" indicates drainage boreholes placed on both sides of the gate roads.

Summary

- To reduce longwall face emissions from the Pittsburgh Coalbed, the most effective borehole pattern is the trilateral configuration (pattern B), followed by the dual-lateral arrangement (pattern A).

- The greatest reduction in methane emissions can be achieved by extending the duration of premining degasification for as long as possible.

- Additional reductions in longwall face methane emissions can be realized by continuing methane drainage during the mining phase.

- The emissions into the gate road entries originate mostly from gas desorbing from the margins of the panel where in-seam, near-margin borehole segments are located.

- Further reductions in methane emissions into the gate roads can be achieved with horizontal methane drainage boreholes on either side of the gate roads, although this method is only applicable to the first panel in a new set. Data for this study are based on the Pittsburgh Coalbed. A more permeable seam may not benefit significantly from the presence of boreholes on either side of the gate road.

3. CHARACTERIZING AND FORECASTING LONGWALL FACE METHANE EMISSION RATES FOR LONGER LONGWALL FACES

This section discusses one of two NIOSH-developed methods for predicting methane emission rates when longwall face lengths increase. The first method by Schatzel et al. [2006] is an adaptation of an earlier NIOSH technique that essentially extrapolates emission rates to longer faces using field monitoring data. The strength of this methodology is in the computation of methane emission rates for each face segment length being mined. A total of eight methane emission rates are shown in the case study. Changing methane emission rates over the length of the longwall face, as well as emissions rate variations over subsequent days, are clearly visible and the causes of these changes are discussed. A second method by Krog et al. [2006] is discussed in Section 4 and is probably better suited to meet the needs of most coal mine operators for forecasting methane emission rates to wider longwall faces. Both methods describe results using the same data set. The two methods produce complementary views of longwall face methane emissions at an operating mine.

Overview

Continuous enhancements in longwall mining equipment have significantly improved face advance rates. This increasing longwall advance rate has generally outpaced the continuous miner gate road advance rates, which had led operators to decrease the relative amount of development mining required by increasing longwall panel sizes, in particular face lengths. The mining of longer longwall faces has the advantage of less development per ton of coal mined on the longwall, but can result in increased methane emissions. Increases in longwall face length can create problems such as increased cumulative face methane emissions and increased potential for methane-related production delays [Krog et al. 2006]. This may be further exacerbated by the complex airflow movements along the face itself. Although airflow movement along the longwall face is generally assumed to be linear, evidence of exchanges between face and gob atmospheres have been noted [Balusu et al. 2001; Wendt and Balusu 2001]. Other researchers have suggested that an increased level of opportunity for air exchanges between face and gob regions result from resistant roof units and associated void spaces behind the longwall face [Noack 1998; Balusu et al. 2001; Wendt and Balusu 2001].

The questions asked by ventilation engineers are: how much of an increase in methane emissions can be expected with the longer longwall face, and how can this increase be mitigated to maintain a safe underground workplace? An increase in the ventilation airflow to dilute the expected increase in methane emissions might not be possible because many modern longwalls are at, or near, their reasonably practical airflow limits. Therefore, the extra methane emissions will generally have to be handled by a combination of increased ventilation airflow, methane drainage, and production management.

Longwall Face Emission Monitoring and Prediction Method

A longwall mine operating in the Pittsburgh Coalbed in southwestern Pennsylvania was studied. The dimensions of the outlined coal block were about 3,250 m (10,700 ft) long by about 315 m (1,030 ft) wide (Figure 13). The study began with 1,250 m (4,100 ft) of panel length remaining. The longwall bleeder system was ventilated by the use of a centrifugal bleeder fan and four vertical gob ventilation boreholes per panel placed at regularly spaced intervals of 610 m (2,000 ft) to provide additional methane control capacity. Four horizontal in-seam methane drainage boreholes were also present adjacent to the gate roads of the study panel [Schatzel et al. 2006].

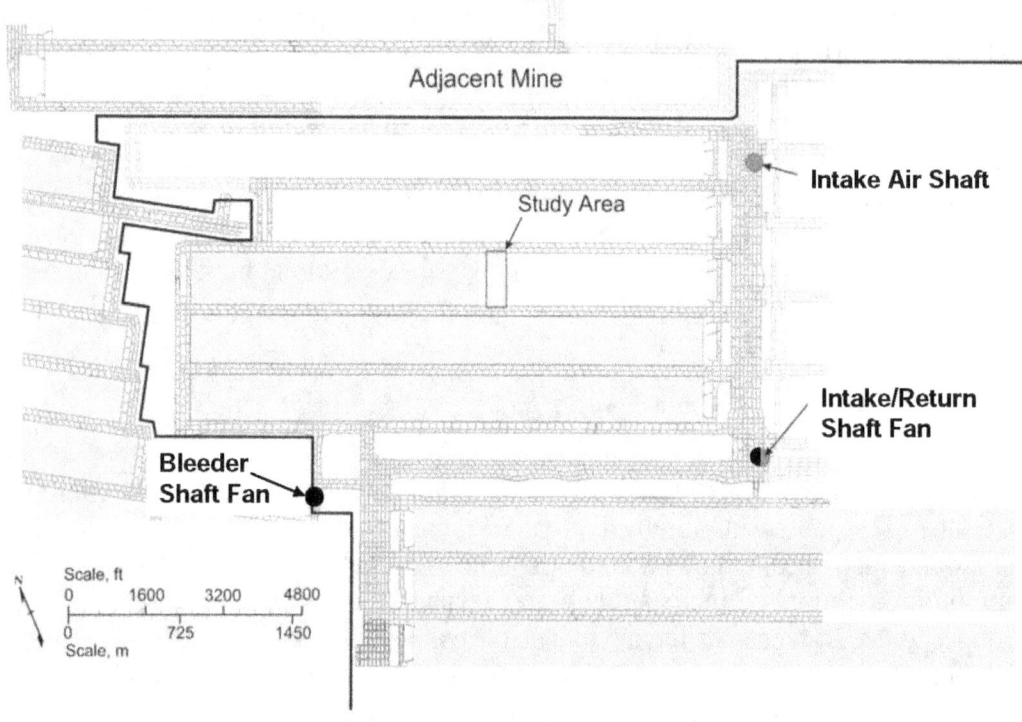

Figure 13.—Longwall face emission study area.

The original methodology for this study was first developed by Diamond and Garcia [1999] to predict methane emission rates for 305-m (1,000-ft) faces based on face emissions monitoring on a 229-m (750-ft) wide face at two adjacent mines operating in the Pocahontas No. 3 Coalbed in Virginia. The face was divided into three equal segments of 76.2 m (250 ft). Average cumulative methane emissions data for each of the three segments were plotted as a function of face length. Curves were fit to the actual emission data and then extrapolated to the 305-m (1,000-ft) face widths to predict methane emission rates on the longer faces.

For this study in the Pittsburgh Coalbed, continuously recording methane monitors were installed along the longwall face. Methane concentrations were recorded by data loggers. Airflow measurements were made at various locations on the face. One shift was monitored on each of the 3 days of the study. A production time study consisting of shearer location on the face (recorded as shield numbers) and shearer mining direction (head-to-tail (H–T) or tail-to-head (T–H)) was conducted throughout the 3 days of the face emissions monitoring [Schatzel et al. 2006; Krog et al. 2006]. In applying this methodology, the following assumptions were made to project methane emissions to longer faces: (1) the mine advance rate and the frequency of mining delays will occur at about the same rate, (2) face methane emissions are assumed to be constant within each segment, (3) all sources of methane emissions change at a constant rate with increased face length, and (4) the solutions are site-specific for the Pittsburgh Coalbed, the ventilation system configuration, and the methane drainage systems applied at the study mine site.

To analyze the movement of methane emissions in the longwall ventilation airflow, the face was divided into four segments of equal length (Figure 14). Methane emission rates were determined for each face segment of each pass of the shearer using the associated methane concentration, ventilation airflow, and time study data. Since the principal focus of this study was longwall face ventilation and methane emissions, the decision was made to position the monitors away from the headgate and tailgate corners to avoid including ventilation air in these areas, which did not traverse the face. The methane sensors were installed at shields 20, 80, and 145 (see "Instrument locations" in Figure 14). On the study panel, belt air was used on the longwall face (Figure 15).

> **Longwall face methane emissions data can be used as the basis for predicting methane emissions on longer longwall faces. An accounting of underground activities near the face is necessary for data analysis. In the methodology described, methane monitors are positioned away from the headgate and tailgate corners to address methane in air moving along the face, not ventilation air losses at the headgate corner or gob gas leakage.**

Characterizing Longwall Face Emissions and Extrapolating Emissions to Longer Faces

A total of 27 methane-related delays were noted during the study. Methane delays were typically of short duration, averaging about 7 min. The belt line made up the great majority of the methane measured at the shield 20 methanometer. Consequently, for analytical purposes, face emissions were assumed to be zero for the first 20 shields of an H–T pass (up to 34 m (114 ft) from the headgate corner) (Figure 15). Methane emissions in this portion of the face were quite low, usually measured as between 0.0 and 0.021 m^3/s (0 and 44 cfm) [Schatzel et al. 2006].

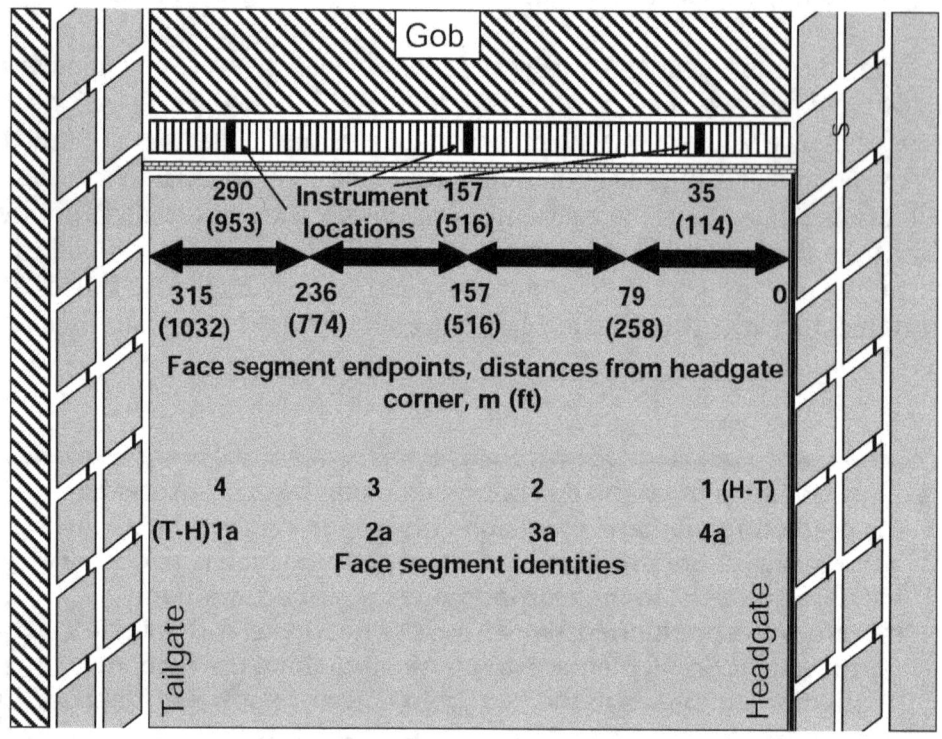

Figure 14.—Pittsburgh Coalbed longwall face emission study site with instrument locations and face segment identities *(not to scale)*.

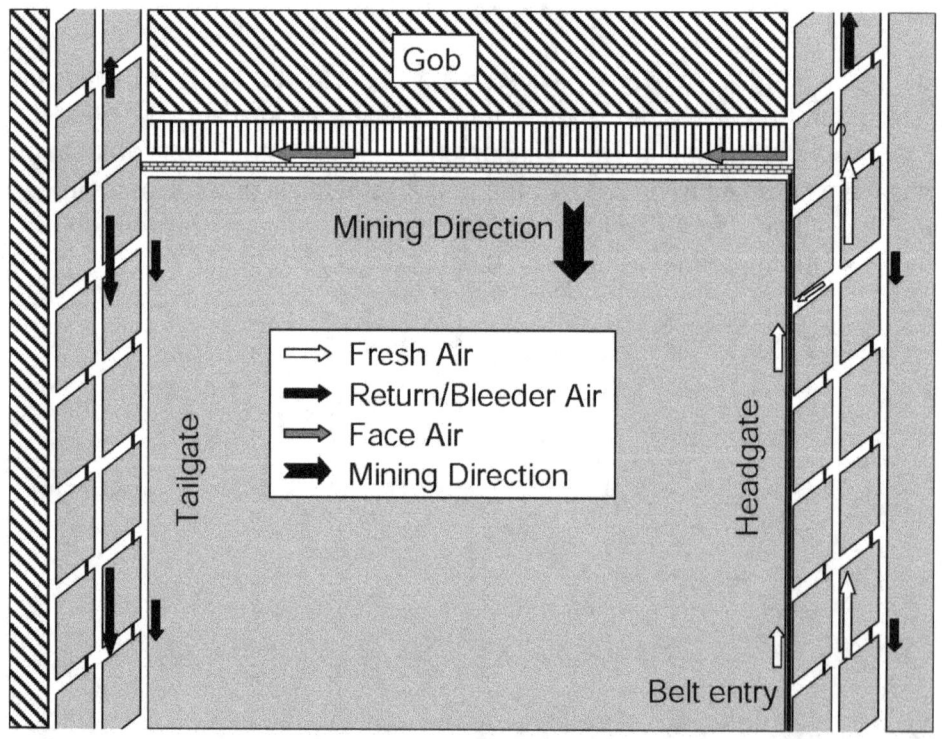

Figure 15.—Ventilation configuration at the study site *(not to scale)*.

The sums of gas emissions from the eight face segments for the H–T and T–H passes were normalized to match actual gas emission totals measured at the shield 145 methane emissions monitor. The cumulative methane emission rates for the face segments for each of the 3 days of the study are shown in Table 6.

> **Face methane emission rates were consistently higher by about 41% in the H–T passes than the T–H passes. This difference in methane emissions rate was caused by the longwall face configuration, which produced a much longer "wedge" cut toward the tailgate side of the face; a slower shearer cutting rate in the T–H passes; and the pan line direction of movement toward the headgate.**

One methane drainage borehole was drilled on each side of the panel. The boreholes were oriented parallel to the gate road entries, 30 m (98 ft) from the respective gate roads (Figure 16). The holes were drilled toward the advancing face, terminating in the study area. Prior to interception by mining, the holes were filled with water so that coalbed gas could not accumulate in the borehole.

Production delays due to increasing methane concentration were most common when the shearer was near the tailgate side of the longwall face of the H–T pass, but began occurring with increasing frequency at locations nearer the headgate side of the face as the study progressed over the 3 days [Schatzel et al. 2006].

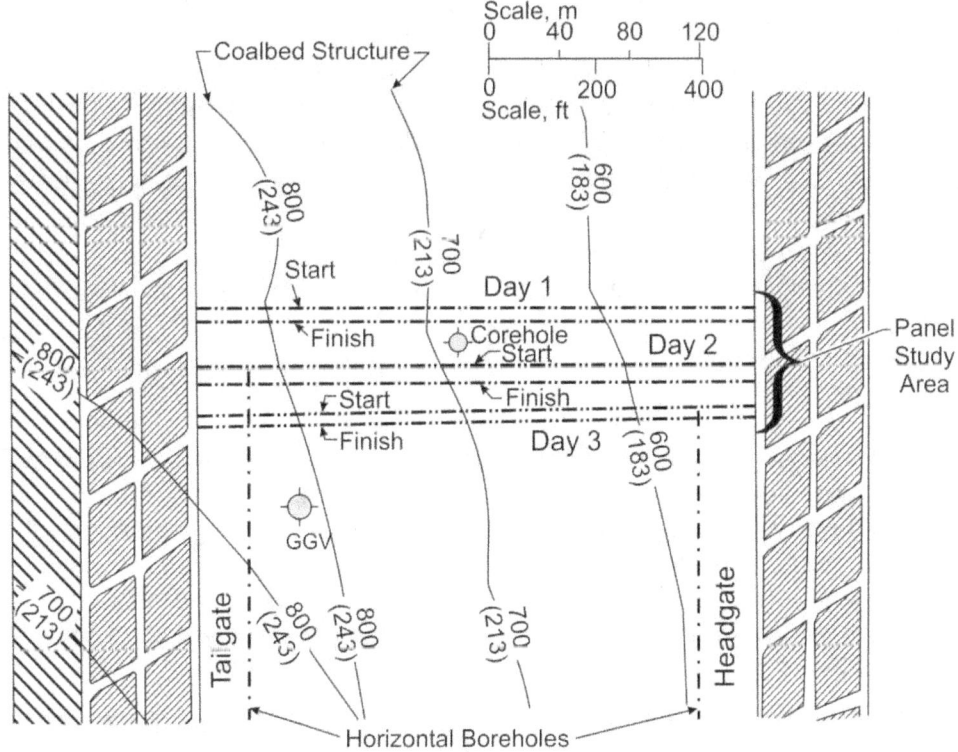

Figure 16.—Actual portions of the study panel monitored for face methane emissions and associated methane drainage borehole locations.

Table 6.—Face segment emission rate data shown for combined averaged H–T, T–H passes

Face segments	Day 1		Day 2		Day 3	
	m³/s	cfm	m³/s	cfm	m³/s	cfm
1, 4a	0.003	7	0.010	20	0.023	49
2, 3a	0.009	18	0.006	13	0.029	61
3, 2a	0.031	66	0.018	37	0.011	24
4, 1a	0.020	42	0.008	18	0.016	33

> **In many mines, the quantity of coalbed methane removed by a gob gas venthole is significant, potentially 75% of the volume of gas emissions on the longwall face. Pressure differentials are also important in defining the flow paths for gas movement. A nearby active gob gas venthole is much more influential than a distant one.**

The variation in emissions behavior can be seen more clearly in Table 6, which shows the average methane emissions from each segment (H–T and T–H combined data) during the 3 days of monitoring (Figure 17). Methane emissions produced during passes on day 1 were relatively low (from 0.003 to 0.009 m³/s (7 to 18 cfm)) in the segments nearest to the headgate (1, 2, 3a, 4a). Emissions increased significantly in segments 3 and 2a (0.031 m³/s (66 cfm)) and diminished somewhat from that level toward the tailgate in segments 4 and 1a. On day 2, methane emission rates in the near-headgate segments 1 and 4a were higher than those on day 1, then decreased in the next segments, 2 and 3a. Similar to day 1, methane emissions increased in face segments 3 and 2a (0.018 m³/s (37 cfm)), then decreased in the face segments toward the tailgate, i.e., face segments 4 and 1a. On day 3, methane emissions were much higher (0.023 m³/s (49 cfm)) near the headgate face segments 1 and 4a than during the prior 2 days of the study (Table 6). The methane emissions rate increased in the next face segments (0.029 m³/s (61 cfm)) 2 and 3a, but then decreased significantly in face segments 3 and 2a (0.011 m³/s (24 cfm)), with a slight increase (0.023 m³/s (49 cfm)) in the tailgate segment face segments 4 and 1a (Figure 17) [Schatzel et al. 2006].

> **Methane delays were most frequent when the shearer was mining near the tailgate. Methane delays on the longwall face increased from the first to third day of the study as the longwall face reached the approximate maximum distance from the nearest operating gob gas venthole prior to interception of the next venthole, 2 days after the study was completed.**

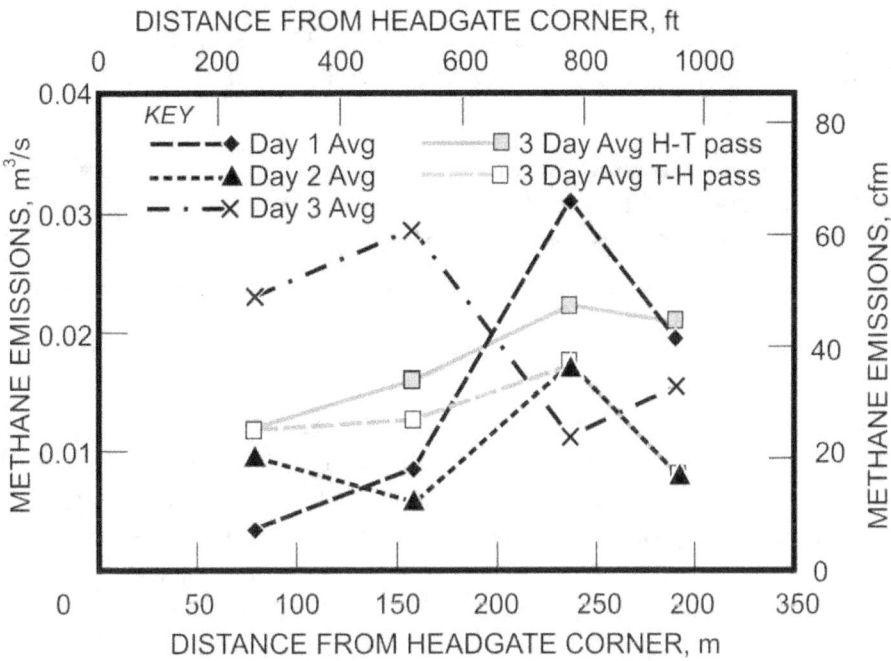

Figure 17.—Average methane emission rates for each day of study determined for each face segment.

On day 2 of the study, the presence of a horizontal borehole on the face was noted near the tailgate side of the panel at shield 140. On day 3 of the study, the interception of the horizontal borehole near the headgate at shield 23 was observed. It is likely that coalbed methane production from the first borehole encountered near shield 140 on the tailgate side of the face had decreased the methane content of the coalbed in the vicinity of the borehole. Consequently, after the borehole was intercepted on day 2 of the study, methane emissions dropped toward the tailgate side, as shown by the comparison of face segments 4 and 1a on day 1 with those on day 2 (Figure 17). A similar drop in methane emission rates was not observed in face segments near the headgate from day 2 and day 3 when the borehole was intercepted near shield 23 (Figure 16). It is not known if methane emissions would have diminished in the region of face segments 1 and 4a if the study had been continued for another day.

> **Methane drainage via horizontal boreholes near the study area seems to be an effective method for reducing longwall face emissions. The variable methane emission characteristics observed on the longwall face were likely produced by emission rate reductions associated with methane drainage boreholes.**

Production delays also affected face methane emission rates. These delays, including those due to high methane emissions, result in lower calculated pass segment methane emission rates because the time to complete the pass segment increases while the longwall face equipment is idle. Therefore, the increased number of methane-related production delays on day 3, and to a lesser extent on day 2, resulted in lower average methane emission rates on some individual pass segments, particularly on tailgate-side face segments 4 and 1a (Figure 17, Table 6). By day 3, methane-related production delays were occurring closer toward the headgate portion of the face, in face segments 3 and 2a, reducing methane emission rates during mining stoppages there as well [Schatzel et al. 2006].

> **Methane-related delays reduce emission rates during face methane monitoring when coal is not being mined.**

Graphs of the cumulative measured average methane emission rates for the ~315-m (~1,030-ft) panel face segments in both the H–T and T–H directions are shown in Figure 18. From these data, two least-squares linear regression curves were calculated to predict methane emissions for longer face lengths of 366, 427, and 488 m (1,200, 1,400, and 1,600 ft) in the Pittsburgh Coalbed. To create trend line A, all H–T and T–H passes were averaged, and then an overall average emission pass plot was created. Trend line A was fit to this overall average emission pass data (Figure 18). The trend line equations are given in metric units. It should be noted that the emission rate for a 315-m (1,030-ft) face is based on a projection of the cumulative emissions data from the face segments projected from shield 145 to shield 157, or 290 m (953 ft) from the headgate corner using data from all of the longwall passes. Trend line B was fit to the H–T passes only. Since most of the delays occurred and higher face methane emission rates occurred on the H–T passes, this plot may be more representative of problematic concentrations of face gas than trend line A, which includes the generally lower T–H pass face emission rate data (Figure 18). Using trend line B, the predicted face methane emissions represent increases of 36%, 61%, and 88% for 366, 426, and 488 m (1,200, 1,400 and 1,600 ft) faces, respectively, compared to the base of about 315-m (1,030-ft) face using all face methane emission data.

> **Since the H–T passes produced higher methane emission rates and more methane concentration delays than the T–H direction, the H–T passes were used to project emission rates to longer faces. In applying this technique, it is recommended that the operator use data from the pass direction, which produced the higher emission rates, to perform the least-squares projection to longer faces.**

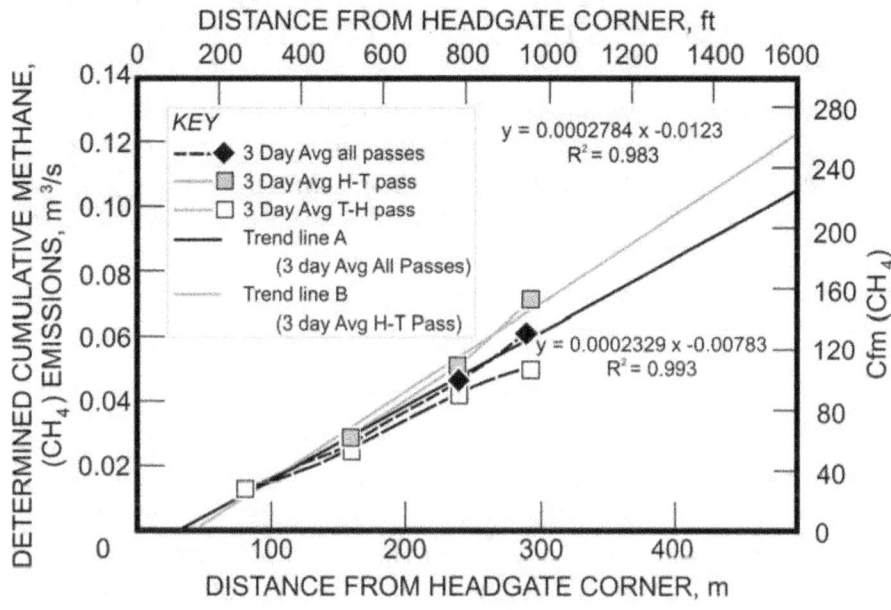

Figure 18.—Methane emission prediction curves for the Pittsburgh Coalbed.

Summary

- Longwall face methane emissions monitoring data can be used as the basis for predicting methane emissions on longer longwall faces.

- The quantity of coalbed methane removed by a GGV is significant, on the order of 70%–75% of gas emissions from the monitored longwall face.

- The tailgate corner continues to challenge ventilation and methane control technology, and most of the methane delays occurred when the shearer was mining near the tailgate.

- Longwall face emissions can be effectively reduced by in-seam, horizontal, methane drainage boreholes. Additional methane drainage techniques applied in advance of mining can also be effective, such as fracked vertical and directionally surface boreholes.

- Face methane emission rates are diminished during methane-related delays and when coal is not being mined.

- In applying this monitoring-based technique for predicting face emissions on longer longwall faces, it is recommended that the operator use data from the pass direction, which produced the higher emission rates.

4. PREDICTING METHANE EMISSIONS FROM LONGER LONGWALL FACES BY ANALYSIS OF EMISSION CONTRIBUTORS

This section describes the second of two methods of longwall face emission prediction techniques. NIOSH conducted a longwall methane emission and mining time study at a mine operating in the Pittsburgh Coalbed to assess the methane emission consequences of mining a longer face. Based on the results of the study, a set of site-specific mathematical formulas and constants were developed to characterize each of four longwall emission contributors. The mathematical formulas were then applied to longer longwall face mining scenarios to predict the methane emissions from these faces.

Overview

A detailed analysis of the methane sources and their individual contributions to the total longwall methane emissions can be obtained from methane concentration data collected at the beginning and end of the longwall face, along with the shearer location and other relevant ventilation and mining data. The methane emission contributors from the mining of a longwall face that were evaluated for this study were (1) gas released from the coal broken by the shearer, (2) gas emitted from the broken coal on the face conveyor, (3) gas emitted from the coal transported on the belt, and (4) background gas emitted from the coal face and adjoining ribs in the intake airway gate road entries. Once the methane contributions from the various sources have been defined for an actual longwall cutting sequence, the methane emissions from an ideal (i.e., delay-free) cut sequence can be predicted. The calculated methane emission contributions can then be extrapolated to longer longwall faces, taking into account the variations in coal production and transport factors, to more accurately predict future methane emission rates from longer longwall faces.

Methodology

This research used the same data set as that described in Section 3. The methane monitors were located at shields 20, 80, and 145 (see "Instrument locations" in Figure 14). These positions were chosen based on previous studies that indicated possible air interactions at the corners of the headgate and tailgate [Diamond and Garcia 1999]. The methane contribution interpretation does not take into account the possible effect of ventilation airflow interactions with the gob, which is consistent with the initial goal of the study [Krog et al. 2006].

The physical aspects, equipment, operational, and ventilation scenarios of the longwall panel (Figure 15) are very important in evaluating methane sources because they determine the mathematical formulas used in the methane contribution model. The site-specific variables for this study are discussed in Krog et al. [2006].

Assumptions

The following assumptions were made:

- Background methane emissions from the longwall face (active, not idle) are linearly dependent on longwall face length.
- Background rib methane emission from the No. 1 belt entry are linearly dependent on the remaining length of the longwall panel, but are independent of longwall face width or activity.
- There is no interaction between the face air and the air in the gob.
- The stage loader located at the headgate was not incorporated in the simulation.
- Methane liberation rate at the shearer is proportional to the cut coal volume.
- Methane liberation rate on the face conveyor is proportional to the product of coal tonnage and elapsed time on the conveyor [Krog et al. 2006].

Construction of Formulas

The following describes the mathematical process used in the evaluation. The longwall face was broken down into 61-m (200-ft) sections to correspond with the width of 30 shields. Since the face conveyor speed was 1.78 m/s (350 ft/min), the transport time for coal over 61 m (200 ft) of the face conveyor was 34 sec (61 m / 1.78 m/s), and the transport time for the counterflowing ventilation airflow was 24 sec (61 m / 2.54 m/s). Therefore, the time for the coal to be transported by the face conveyor and the time required for the counterflowing air to transit the same distance adds up to 58 sec, which was rounded to 1 min to match the methane concentration readings being recorded every minute. The emission times for methane from the sources of interest, as well as transit times for the associated ventilation airflows, can be summarized as follows:

- Coal cut by shearer, 0–2 min
- Coal on face conveyor, 1–3 min
- Airflow along longwall face, 2 min
- Coal on belt, 5 min
- Airflow along belt, 10 min

When the shearer is cutting coal, the liberation of methane from the coal face will be recorded by the methane monitor located near the tailgate at shield 145, either instantly or up to 2 min later, depending on the shearer's location. When the shearer is located on the tailgate side of shield 145, no extra methane liberated by the shearer will be recorded by the methane monitor. If the shearer is located within 61 m (200 ft) on the headgate side of shield 145, then methane liberation due to the cutting of the coal will be recorded for that minute. When the coal was cut nearer the headgate, it would take up to 2 min for the face air to travel to the methane sensor located at shield 145.

The contribution of methane emissions from the coal on the face conveyor is more complicated than the above circumstances because coal cut by the shearer can be transported on the face conveyor for 1–3 min. To determine the transport time for methane emissions from the coal on the face conveyor, the counterflowing longwall ventilation airflow and the shearer

39

location/direction of travel must be taken into account. For example, coal cut at shield 145 will release methane that will be recorded at shield 145 instantly (0 min). Coal transported on the face conveyor will release gas into the face ventilation airflow for a total of 3 min (0–2 min), during which time the counterflowing face ventilation will take up to 2 min to reach shield 145. Therefore, methane emitted from the coal on the face conveyor will be recorded at shield 145 for 0–4 min in this example.

> **If a methane delay is triggered by a methane monitor's high methane reading, the underlying increase in methane emissions may have occurred several minutes earlier. To reduce methane-related production delays, an understanding of methane emission sources and their magnitudes is required.**

Continuing this example, methane emissions from the coal on the belt will be recorded at shield 145 for 5–19 min after coal was initially cut at shield 145 (2 min for the face conveyor, 2 min for the face airflow transit time, 1–5 min for the belt transport time, and 0–10 min for the belt airflow transit time). Therefore, coal mechanically cut by the shearer will affect methane emission levels near the tailgate instantly and for as long as 19 min after being cut [Krog et al. 2006].

The contributions of methane from individual sources over time has led to a simple set of five linear equations for shearer, face conveyor, belt, background emissions from the coal face, and background emissions from the adjoining ribs in the intake gate roads, which were solved for each minute of the three shifts monitored. Constants in each equation were calculated by least-squares linear regression such that the calculated results best matched the actual readings at shields 20 and 145.

Results

The calculated emission constants were consistent for the 3 days of the study, except for the background methane levels at shield 20. This value varied considerably over the 3 days of the study. The reason for the observed dramatic increase in this value is most likely the interception of a horizontal degas hole located upwind of the shield 20 methane sensor [Schatzel et al. 2006]. After considering the consistency of the emission constants for the other three components (face conveyor, belt, and shearer) from shields 20 and 145 individually and combined, it was decided to use the 3-day average for shields 20 and 145 for further evaluation of the background emission component [Krog et al. 2006].

Table 7 shows the calculated average methane emission rates for each contributor using the daily constants for shields 20 and 145. The "total" values in the table are the calculated average methane for the individual days. The "actual" values are the recorded methane for the individual days.

Table 7.—Daily methane emission contributor averages and percentages using daily shield 20 and 145 constants

Shield 20 and 145 Daily results	Conveyor (m^3/s)	Belt (m^3/s)	Shearer (m^3/s)	Face (m^3/s)	Rib (m^3/s)	Total (m^3/s)	Actual (m^3/s)
Day 1	0.012	0.015	0.005	0.027	−0.001	0.057	0.057
Day 2	0.005	0.014	0.004	0.028	0.002	0.052	0.052
Day 3	0.007	0.006	0.005	0.030	0.019	0.068	0.068
Average	0.008	0.012	0.005	0.029	0.006	0.059	0.059

Shield 20 and 145 Daily results	Conveyor (cfm)	Belt (cfm)	Shearer (cfm)	Face (cfm)	Rib (cfm)	Total (cfm)	Actual (cfm)
Day 1	26	31	10	57	−3	121	121
Day 2	11	29	8	60	3	111	111
Day 3	15	14	11	64	40	143	143

Shield 20 and 145 Daily results	Conveyor (%)	Belt (%)	Shearer (%)	Face (%)	Rib (%)	Total (%)	Actual (%)
Day 1	22%	26%	8%	47%	−3%	100%	100%
Day 2	10%	26%	7%	54%	3%	100%	100%
Day 3	10%	9%	8%	45%	28%	100%	100%
Average	14%	20%	8%	49%	9%	100%	100%

Table 8.—Methane contribution percentages from longwall emission contributors during gas delays compared to daily averages for a 315-m (1,030-ft) longwall face

Methane contributions		Conveyor	Belt	Shearer	Background
3-day averages		17%	19%	6%	59%

Gas delays	No.				
Cutting gas delays	23	32%	18%	9%	42%
H–T gas delays	19	33%	18%	9%	41%
T–H gas delays	4	26%	18%	8%	48%

The face and rib emissions represent about 59% of the total daily emissions; however, this percentage is somewhat misleading because these emissions continue throughout the entire shift, even during mining delays. In contrast, the shearer, face conveyor, and belt emissions are intermittent sources (i.e., they are only a factor during active mining on the face and during coal transport), but they are the primary contributors to longwall face gas delays, as shown in Table 8.

The calculated methane contributions clearly show that the H–T passes experience higher methane concentrations than the T–H passes [Krog et al. 2006]. The time study data for the 3 days of the study showed 19 gas delays (shutdowns of mining equipment due to excessive methane concentrations) on 10 of the 11 complete H–T passes. The average location for the gas delays on the H–T passes was shield 119, 245 m (804 ft) or 78% of the distance from the headgate corner.

41

Monitoring data show that when longwall gas delays occur, the methane contributions from the face conveyor and shearer dramatically increase in their relative contribution to the total face emissions. Controlling these two emission sources is critical to maintaining statutory limits at the working face and avoiding methane emission-related coal production delays.

There were four gas delays recorded on three of the nine T–H passes. The average location for the gas delays on the T–H passes was shield 71, 146 m (480 ft) or 46% of the distance down the longwall face from the headgate corner [Krog et al. 2006].

The direction of cutting affects methane emissions on the longwall face because at the end of an H–T pass, the face conveyor, shearer, and belt are all contributing gas at or near their maximum rate. The T–H passes do not have coincidental maximums for face conveyor, shearer, and belt emissions, so a more consistent emission rate occurs over the entire cut sequence. This explains the less frequent gas delays on T–H passes. Of the 11 H–T passes over the three shifts that were monitored for this study, only one cut did not have a gas delay, but it did have a face conveyor delay. A total of 10 complete passes had gas delays. Of the nine T–H passes, three had gas delays.

Figure 19 shows the calculated methane contributor components for day 1 using the 3-day average constants of shields 20 and 145. The calculated methane contribution is the product of the 3-day average constants of shields 20 and 145 and the formula results for each minute for day 1. Additional analyses and graphs of the data are presented by Krog et al. [2006].

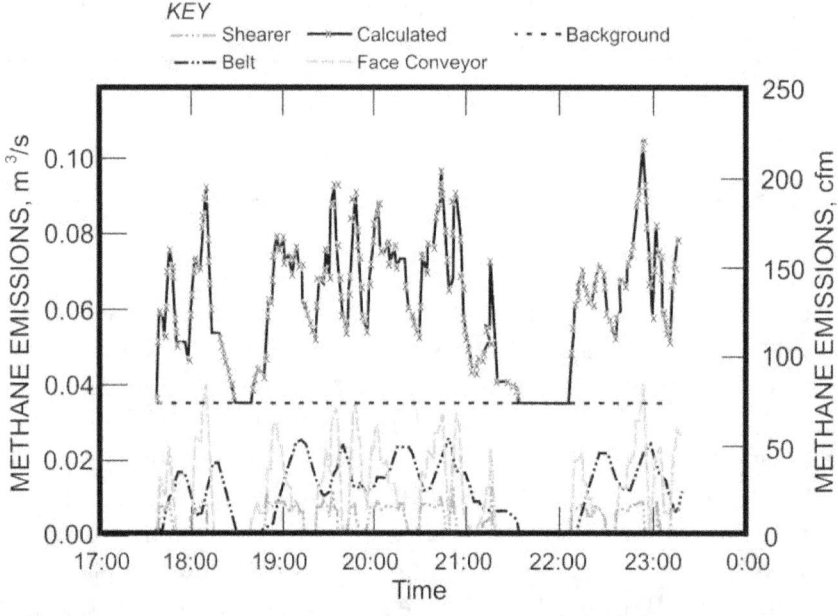

Figure 19.—Calculated individual methane contributors and total calculated methane emissions for study day 1.

> **Analysis of face methane emission rates indicates that gas delays occurred during periods of high emissions. The predictive emissions provided good correlation between the measured and predicted methane emission rates during the delays.**

Technique for Predicting Methane Emissions on Longer Longwall Faces

Coal production and transport factors have an important influence on overall methane emission rates on the longwall face. Coal productivity (coal volume mined per hour) will be increased for a longer face since the cut cycles are face length-dependent. At longer face lengths, the wedge/sumping times are assumed to be the same as those for the base case, but the cutting times will increase proportionally to the face length, minus the sumping distance.

Assuming that the longwall face conveyor can keep up with the shearer and the shearer cuts at the same speed over the greater face length, it follows that the productivity of the shearer will increase because a greater percentage of time will be allotted to cutting than sumping. Therefore, the total methane liberation from the mined coal during a shift would increase, but the shearer's emission rate during cutting will remain the same for a longer longwall face if the cutting speed remains constant. The rib emission will be linearly dependent on the remaining length of the panel. The background emissions for the longwall face will increase linearly with face length. However, if the belt line is used as a source of face air, the background emission from the intake rib will remain constant.

The face conveyor, if operating at a constant speed, will transport a greater volume of coal per hour for a longer longwall face. The face conveyor will also transport the coal over a greater distance and for a longer time, thereby increasing the methane emissions from this component on a longer longwall face. The belt emissions are a function of the amount of coal on the belt, the transport time, and the amount and direction of belt air. The belt emissions can also reach a steady-state maximum when the entire belt is full with coal, thereby capping the upper limit of belt emissions regardless of panel width [Krog et al. 2006].

> **The expected peak methane emission increases for wider longwall panels result primarily from the coal transported on the face conveyor and the background emissions from the larger area of exposed coal on the face. Methane emissions associated with the cutting of coal on the face by the shearer will remain constant for longer longwall face lengths as long as the cutting speed remains constant.**

The calculated results for methane emissions on longer longwall faces are predicted for a location 15 m (50 ft) outby the tailgate corner before any possible interaction with the gob gas near the tailgate. For a 305-m (1,000-ft) wide longwall panel, methane emissions were predicted for two full cuts without delays. The predicted peak methane emission of 0.110 m^3/s (234 cfm) closely matches the maximum values recorded during the study—0.099 m^3/s (210 cfm) [Krog et al. 2006]. Figure 20 shows the predicted methane emissions for two full cuts without any delays for a 488-m (1,600-ft) wide longwall panel. The calculated peak methane emissions for the 488-m (1,600-ft) wide longwall panel are 37% higher than for the roughly 305-m (1,000-ft) wide longwall panel.

Coal on the face conveyor caused the largest calculated increase in methane emission rates on the longer longwall faces, whereas coal cut by the shearer and on the belt, as expected, caused no increase (Table 9). The face conveyor's methane emission increase is due to the increased length and time that the coal will be carried by the conveyor. Keeping the length of the remaining panel (and thus the length of the belt) constant at 1,195 m (3,920 ft) for each of the increased face length emission calculations precludes any extra peak methane load being emitted by coal on the belt.

> **Two methods exist for reducing longwall face methane concentrations produced by all sources. The first is to increase the amount of face airflow. Second, long-term methane drainage will also reduce the methane contents in the coal, thereby reducing methane emissions from potentially all methane contributors.**

Table 9.—Calculated rates for methane emission contributors on idealized passes on longer longwall faces

Face width (m)	Conveyor (m^3/s)	Belt (m^3/s)	Shearer (m^3/s)	Background (m^3/s)	Peak (m^3/s)
305	0.040	0.027	0.009	0.035	0.110
366	0.048	0.027	0.009	0.040	0.124
427	0.056	0.027	0.009	0.046	0.138
488	0.064	0.027	0.009	0.052	0.152
Face width (ft)	Conveyor (cfm)	Belt (cfm)	Shearer (cfm)	Background (cfm)	Peak (cfm)
1,000	85	58	18	73	234
1,200	101	58	18	86	263
1,400	118	58	18	98	292
1,600	135	58	18	110	322
Percent relative to 305-m (1,000-ft) longwall face					
Face width	Conveyor	Belt	Shearer	Background	Peak
305 m (1,000 ft)	100%	100%	100%	100%	100%
366 m (1,200 ft)	120%	100%	100%	117%	112%
427 m (1,400 ft)	140%	100%	100%	134%	125%
488 m (1,600 ft)	160%	100%	100%	150%	137%

The background emissions increase with longer face lengths because of the increase in exposed longwall face area. However, the methane contribution from the gate road ribs does not increase because the length of the gate roads remains constant in these calculations. It should also be noted that the longer longwall faces will theoretically have higher coal productivity because a greater percentage of time will be spent cutting coal instead of sumping [Krog et al. 2006].

As mentioned previously, the highest predicted methane emissions for longer longwall faces are near the end of the H–T cuts, when the emissions from the coal on the face conveyor and belt are at their highest (Table 9). During the three shifts monitored for this study, 1 of the 11 complete H–T passes did not have a gas delay, but it did have a face conveyor delay. Slowing down the shearer for the second half of the face traverse will reduce the peak methane emissions and give a more consistent emission level. The influence of shearer cutting speed on emissions for the 488-m (1,600-ft) panel is shown graphically in Figure 21. The figure depicts face methane emission rates for the shearer traveling at 14 m/min (50 ft/min) for the first 250 m (820 ft) of the H–T cuts, then at 12 m/min (39 ft/min), and finally at 10 m/min (33 ft/min) to the tailgate.

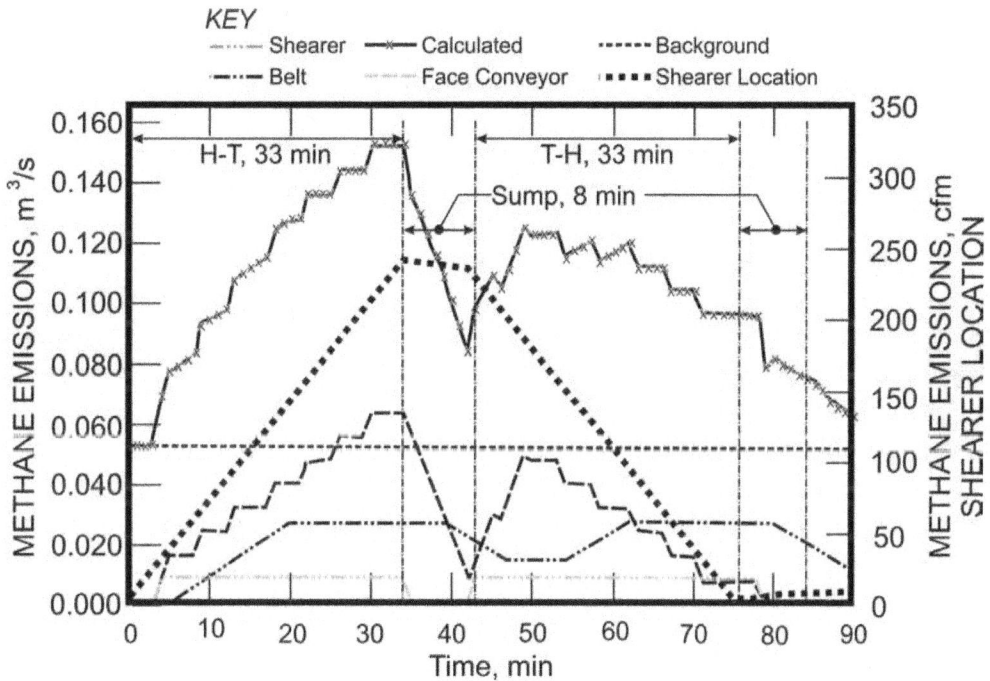

Figure 20.—Calculated methane emissions for two full cuts without delays for a 488-m (1,600-ft) longwall face.

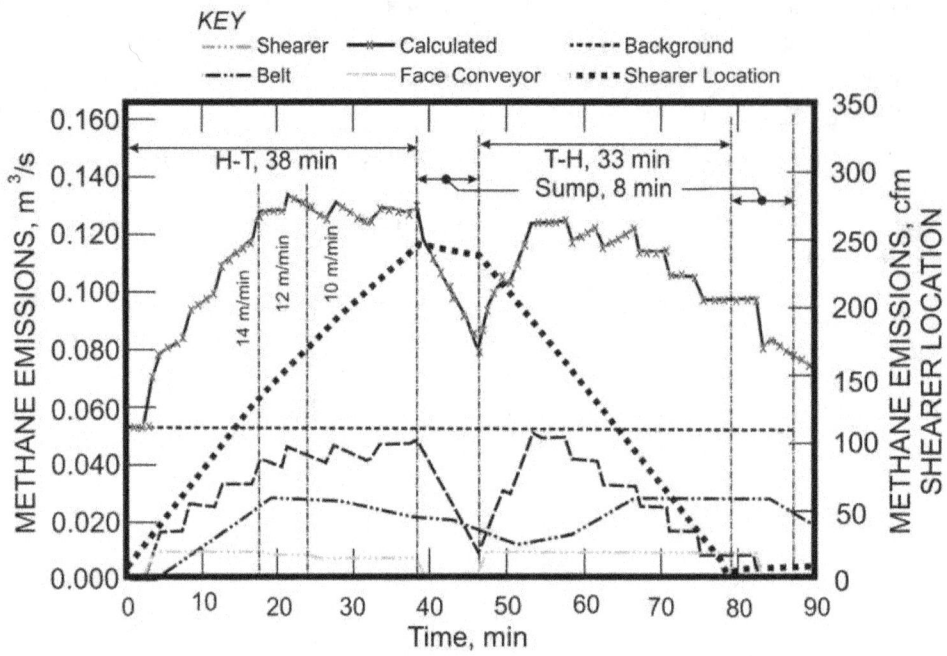

Figure 21.—Calculated influence of variable shearer transit speed pass for a 488-m (1,600-ft) longwall face.

The reduction in methane emission rates resulting from slowing the shearer cutting speed is dramatic, with only 86% (0.131/0.152/ m³/s (278/322 cfm)) of the peak methane emissions being encountered. The 5 extra minutes required to cut the H–T pass due to the reduced shearer transit time (Figure 21) is still less than the observed average gas delay of 7 min for H–T passes. By slowing the shearer cutting speed on H–T passes, the calculated peak methane emission values based on the cutting direction are now within 7% of each other, compared to the 20% difference for the full-speed H–T pass (Figures 20–21).

The conversion of the belt entry to return airflow and the conversion of the No. 3 return entry to intake could increase total airflow at the longwall face, as well as eliminate the belt coal methane emission component from the total methane emission load reaching the tailgate corner of the face. The primary drawback to this conversion is that the No. 3 entry ribs tend to have a higher background methane emission rate than that of the No. 1 entry ribs due to the virgin coal along the No. 3 entry's rib.

> **Mine operators have several options to reduce or dilute methane emissions expected from wider longwall panels:**
>
> 1. **Increasing ventilation airflow quantities to the longwall face**
> 2. **Reducing the shearer transit speed, especially on H–T passes**
> 3. **Using or increasing methane drainage techniques to reduce emissions from all the considered sources by reducing the methane content of the coal**
> 4. **Implementing ventilation design changes, e.g., not coursing the belt entry's ventilation airflow to the face**

Summary

- High methane emission rates may have occurred minutes before their detection and response by sensors.

- Methane contributions from the face conveyor and shearer dramatically increase in their relative contribution to the total face emissions during gas delays.

- Peak methane emission increases for wider longwall panels will result primarily from the coal transported on the face conveyor and the background emissions from face coal.

- Mine operators have several options to reduce or dilute methane emissions expected from wider longwall panels:

  1. Increasing ventilation airflow quantities to the longwall face
  2. Reducing the shearer transit speed, especially on II–T passes
  3. Using or increasing methane drainage techniques
  4. Implementing ventilation design changes

5. DEVELOPMENT OF NUMERICAL MODELS TO INVESTIGATE PERMEABILITY CHANGES, DISTRIBUTIONS, AND GAS EMISSIONS AROUND A LONGWALL PANEL

Overview

Once a longwall face begins retreating, the formation of the longwall gob begins. Underground longwall mining of coal causes disturbance of the overlying rock mass. The caved rock (gob) behind the retreating longwall face can contain high void ratios, providing high permeability flow paths to the methane. The disturbance can increase the rock mass permeability through a reduction on the stress, as well as formation of new fractures in the rock. Methane gas contained in the disturbed rock mass can migrate toward the low-pressure mine workings and present an explosion hazard. This section describes the application of a finite-difference program to predict permeability changes within the rock mass using empirical relationships between fracture permeability and stress.

The extent of rock failure is determined using a geomechanical model that considers both rock matrix and bedding plane failure. The caved rock (gob) is modeled as a compressible, granulated material. The calculated two-dimensional horizontal and vertical permeabilities around the longwall face are averaged and used as one of the inputs to the reservoir model. The modeling approach provides a basis for estimating methane inflow and optimizing control measures. The reservoir simulator models methane desorption from the coal matrix, methane release from the rock layers, and flow toward the mine excavations. The reservoir model was calibrated against records of methane flow at a study mine in southwestern Pennsylvania. Good correlation between actual gas production and model outputs has been achieved [Esterhuizen and Karacan 2005].

This section also describes a newly developed methodology to determine both horizontal and vertical variations in the permeability of the gob. Estimating the permeability distribution within the gob poses challenges due to its complexity. Variations of the permeability in the vertical direction are based on a model of caving and block rotation, which considers the effect of block dimensions and fall height on the void ratio. Gob compaction by the overburden and associated permeability changes are determined from a three-dimensional (3-D) geomechanical model, which simulates the gob as a strain-hardening granular material. The resulting 3-D permeability distribution in the gob is then transferred to a reservoir model. This section demonstrates the application of the method and shows that reasonable results are obtained when compared to empirical experience and measurements [Esterhuizen and Karacan 2007].

Model Development

A two-staged approach has been followed to develop models of methane emissions and flow around longwall mines. The first stage has been to make use of the Itasca Consulting Group's [2000] FLAC2D (Fast Lagrangian Analysis of Continua) finite difference code to simulate the geomechanical response of the rock mass to longwall mining. The program was used to calculate the stress changes, extent of rock fracturing, and bedding plane shear. The output of the FLAC models was used to calculate likely permeability changes based on empirical relationships. The permeability distribution was then used to develop inputs for the 3-D Generalized Equation-of-State Model (GEM) compositional reservoir simulator by Computer

Modelling Group [2003]. The reservoir simulator was used to develop a model of several longwall panels in a study mine against which the model was calibrated by history matching of GGV methane production. The model has been used to evaluate the relative merits of methane drainage options.

Permeabilities measured by Hasenfus et al. [1988] in strata above the Pittsburgh Coalbed demonstrated that the permeability can vary by several orders of magnitude in different sections of a vertical borehole. Hasenfus et al. measured hydraulic conductivities of 7×10^{-6} cm/s (3×10^{-6} in/s) in sandstone near the ground surface. Brutcher et al. [1990] tested the conductivity of a sandstone aquifer and found the values to vary between 10^{-4} and 10^{-6} cm/s (10^{-4} and 10^{-6} in/s) while shale conductivity was one order of magnitude lower. Booth and Spande [1992] reported hydraulic conductivities of 9×10^{-5} cm/s (4×10^{-5} in/s) for sandstone in southern Illinois. Matetic et al. [1995] reported permeabilities of 7×10^{-6} cm/s (3×10^{-6} in/s) in shale materials near surface and 7×10^{-5} cm/s (3×10^{-5} in/s) for sandstone in southeastern Ohio.

The field-measured hydraulic conductivities all fall within published ranges for sandstones and shales, and the upper limits fall within the range that one would expect for jointed rock. Coal measure rocks in the Eastern United States are typically poorly jointed but contain bedding planes that act as discontinuities, which allow horizontal flow. Vertical flow is constrained, especially by thin clay layers. Changes in stress can produce large variations in the permeability of laboratory- and field-scale rock. The permeability of the field-scale rock mass is affected by the closure or opening of fractures under changing stresses. The equivalent permeability can be related to the fracture aperture and fracture spacing [Bai and Elsworth 1993; Hoek and Bray 1981; Louis 1969]. In addition to stress changes, fracturing occurs in the rock mass in the vicinity of a longwall panel. Three zones can be distinguished in the roof rocks: the caved zone, fractured zone, and bending zone [Peng and Chiang 1984; Singh and Kendorski 1981].

FLAC2D models were used to simulate rock behavior along a longitudinal section through the centerline and a section across the width of a typical longwall panel at the study mine. The longitudinal sections were used to assess stress changes and rock failure around the advancing longwall face. The cross-section was used to assess rock behavior around the edges of the longwall, which included the behavior over the chain pillars left between longwall panels. The model dimensions were typically 400 m (1,300 ft) wide by 350 m (1,150 ft) deep to simulate a longitudinal section through a longwall panel [Esterhuizen and Karacan 2005].

Rock Permeability Calculations

Permeability changes were calculated for both stress changes and rock fracturing. Permeabilities were calculated independently for the horizontal and vertical directions. Equations 3 and 4 were used to determine the stress-affected horizontal and vertical permeabilities, respectively:

$$K_h = K_{h0} \times e^{-0.25(\sigma_{yy} - \sigma_{yy0})} \tag{3}$$

$$K_v = K_{v0} \times e^{-0.25(\sigma_{xx} - \sigma_{xx0})} \tag{4}$$

where K is permeability, σ_{xx} and σ_{yy} are the horizontal and vertical stresses, and the "0" subscript indicates initial conditions [Esterhuizen and Karacan 2005].

The permeability of fractured rock was determined from published values of jointed rock and fractured rocks [Hoek and Bray 1981]. Model elements that fail in compression are assumed to experience an increase in permeability of 100 md above their current permeability in both the horizontal and vertical directions, regardless of rock type. Similarly bedding shear failure is assumed to increase the permeability by 50 md in the bedding (horizontal) direction. The fracture- and shear-related permeability changes are added to the current permeabilities at the time of failure. The new permeability is then subject to further variation as a result of stress changes using the logic described above.

The gob is formed by rock fragments that fall from the roof strata into the void created by the removal of the coalbed. The bulking of the gob is affected by the fall height of the rock fragments as well as the size and shape of the fragments. When the fall height is greater than the lateral dimension of the rock fragments, they are more likely to rotate and come to rest in a jumble, which produces relatively large void spaces. As caving proceeds upward, the caved rock occupies an ever-increasing proportion of the free space, thus reducing the fall height of the subsequent fragments. As the fall height reduces, the potential for fragments to rotate diminishes and the amount of bulking is reduced.

The variation of the bulking of the gob in the vertical direction was estimated using a procedure suggested by Munson and Nenzley [1980]. The procedure assumes that maximum bulking of the caved rock will occur when the fall height exceeds about twice the block width. The maximum bulking factor was assumed to be 75% after tests on simulated gob materials [Pappas and Mark 1993]. The bulking factor (S) is expressed as

$$S = \frac{V_r + V_v}{V_r}$$

(5)

where V_r is the rock volume and V_v is the void volume. It was further assumed that a smooth transition will occur from the maximum bulking factor to zero when the fall height is zero [Esterhuizen and Karacan 2007].

The resulting variation in the bulking factor with vertical distance above the floor of a 1.8-m (6-ft) high coalbed was calculated using this relationship for various block widths. Near the floor of the mined coalbed, the bulking factor remains at about 75%, but there is a rapid drop in the bulking factor at about 2.7–4.6 m (9–15 ft) above the floor, depending on the block width. This lower zone is known as the fully caved zone; the upper zone is the partially caved zone.

The effect of gob compaction by the weight of the overlying strata was introduced by assuming the bulking factor will reduce in direct proportion to the amount of compaction. For example, 10% compaction will reduce the bulking factor by 10% of the current value at all points, regardless of the distance above the coalbed floor. This is a simplifying assumption, which does not significantly affect the permeability results.

The Carman-Kozeny equation for flow-through porous media was used to estimate the permeability of the gob (K) as follows:

$$K = \frac{K_0}{0.241} \left(\frac{n^3}{(1-n)^2} \right)$$

(6)

where K_0 is the base permeability of the broken rock at the maximum porosity, and n is the porosity. The value of K_0 was taken as 1×10^6 md, which places it in the "open jointed rock" range according to Hoek and Bray [1981]. This permeability value also falls within the same range of permeabilities calculated from experimental friction factors for flow-through crushed stone compiled by Stephenson [1979]. The K_0 value of 1×10^6 md results in realistic GGV production when used in reservoir modeling of longwalls [Karacan et al. 2007b].

The results indicate that the permeability is 1×10^6 md in the lower part of the gob, where bulking is at the maximum. This high-permeability zone extends to about 1.5 times the mining height. The permeability rapidly decreases at points that are more than about 3 m (10 ft) above floor. The permeability soon drops to 100 md at a height of about 6.1–9.1 m (20–30 ft), which places it in the permeability range of jointed rock. This height corresponds with the empirical observation that cave rock extends about four to six times the height of the mined coalbed [Mucho et al. 2000].

Distribution of Gob Permeability in a Mined Panel

The compaction of the gob behind the longwall face and the associated permeability changes were determined through the use of the FLAC3D numerical modeling program [Itasca Consulting Group 2005]. The program allowed realistic modeling of stress redistribution about a longwall panel and was able to model rock fracture and gob compaction. The gob was modeled using the double-yield material type in FLAC3D, which represented materials in which there may be significant irreversible compaction in addition to shear yielding. The material parameters were selected to simulate a gob material that has an initial bulking factor of 0.75, displaying an exponential increase in load as it is compacted by the weight of the overlying strata. Further details of the modeling approach and typical input parameters are presented by Esterhuizen and Karacan [2005].

> **Permeability varies considerably within the gob. Near the edges of the gob, model results show that the permeability is relatively high, with a maximum of 1×10^6 md estimated near the corners of the mined panel. The permeability in the central part of the gob seems to be relatively constant at about 1×10^5 md. These values are most meaningful for mines operating in the Pittsburgh Coalbed.**

The FLAC3D model can be set up to simulate the progressive extraction of coal by a retreating longwall panel. The void behind the face and the roof rocks up to four to six times the mining height are filled with gob material. The overburden rocks in the model will subside and compact the gob until a state of equilibrium is reached. The compaction of the gob was obtained by querying the FLAC3D model at selected points. Knowing the compaction distribution, it was possible to calculate the remaining void space at each point. It was then a matter of calculating the porosity and associated permeability values using the Carman-Kozeny equation. It was assumed that the horizontal permeability was twice the vertical permeability owing to the shape of rock fragments.

> **The data show that the typical gob gas venthole locations near the tailgate margin of the panel, in this case a distance of about 90 m (300 ft), are well-positioned to intersect the higher permeability zones above the gob.**

Summary

- Permeability values determined for the gob decrease from the margin of the gob to the center of the gob by about a factor of 10 to about 1×10^5 md.

- The design of GGVs should include the interception of the higher permeability zone near the tailgate gate road.

6. METHANE EMISSION CONTROL DURING MINING OF LONGWALL PANELS USING GOB GAS VENTHOLES

Overview

The caving of material filling in the void space formed by the removal of the extracted coalbed and the induced fracturing into the mine roof and floor produce an extensive, voluminous coalbed methane reservoir. The coalbed methane accumulating in the growing gob soon becomes the largest single gas source in the underground mining environment when using the longwall mining method [Curl 1978; Schatzel et al. 1992]. Although ventilation pressure differentials on the active panel are maintained to keep the gob gas from accumulating on the longwall face, gob gas typically contributes to the coalbed gas concentrations at the tailgate side of the face. The longwall gob gas can also contribute to gas accumulations in the gate roads and bleeder system.

High methane emissions originating from the active face areas and from the fractured formations overlying and underlying the mined coalbed can adversely affect both safety and productivity in underground coal mines. Since ventilation alone may not be sufficient to control the methane levels in the longwall mining environment, GGVs have become a standard supplementary methane control option in many mines. These ventholes intercept and capture gas released from the subsided strata before it can enter the ventilation system, thus reducing emissions into the mine entries.

Background

The recovery of methane from longwall gob areas requires consideration of both rock mechanics and fluid dynamics principles in the context that gas flow through strata is mainly controlled by the permeability of the rock units involved. This in turn is a function of the stress disturbances caused by mining activity. To improve gas capture at a reasonable cost, it is important to understand the behavior of the entire GGV system, including the venthole placement and completion strategies, and the reservoir properties of the gob. In order to investigate the effect of GGV completion parameters, a typical multipanel longwall mine was modeled using Computer Modelling Group's [2003] GEM.

The mine selected for this study operates in the Pittsburgh Coalbed in Greene County, Pennsylvania. Overburden depths in the area range between 150 and 270 m (500 and 900 ft). Longwall panels in the old mining districts of this mine were 253 m (830 ft) wide and were increased to about 305 m (1,000 ft). The alteration of permeability fields in and above the panels as a result of the mining-induced disturbances has been estimated from mechanical modeling of the overlying rock mass using FLAC [Itasca Consulting Group 2000]. Model calibration was performed through history-matching the gas production from GGVs in the study area. Figure 22 shows the 3-D grid model that was constructed for this study. The figure shows only the Waynesburg Coalbed (top layer) and Pittsburgh Coalbed (bottom layer). The other layers between the Waynesburg and Pittsburgh Coalbeds have been removed for a better visualization of the wellbores used in the model [Karacan et al. 2006].

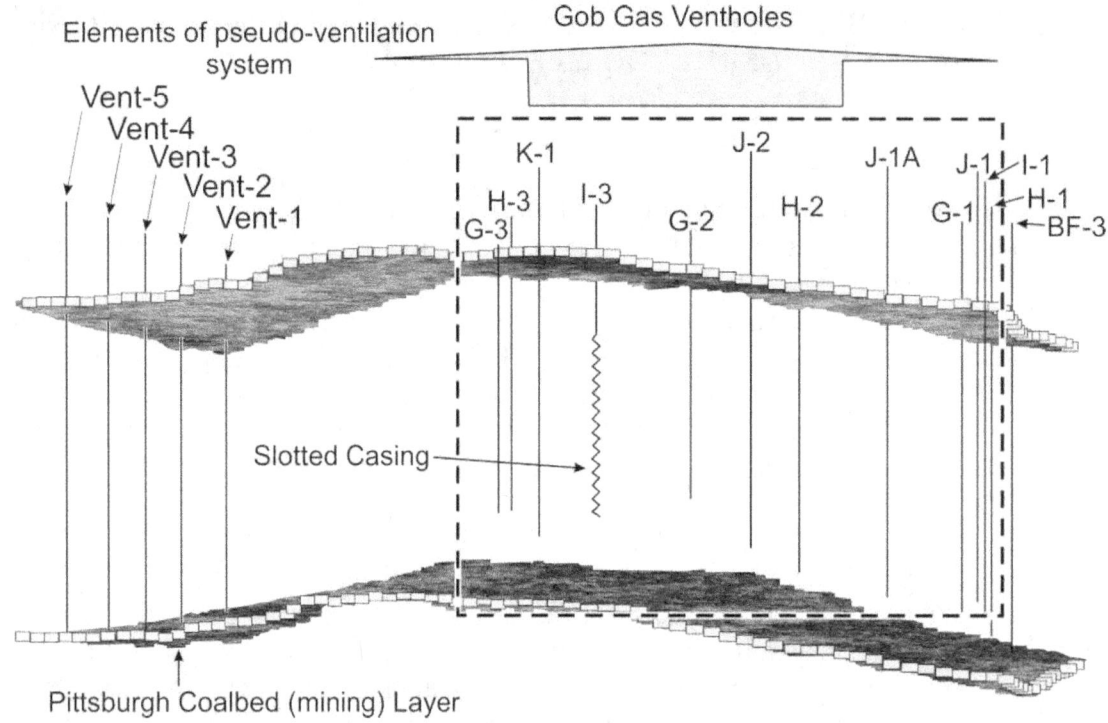

Figure 22.—Three-dimensional representation of grid model of the study area that shows the Waynesburg _(top layer)_ and Pittsburgh _(bottom layer)_ Coalbeds. Also shown are GGVs, their placement, completion representation, and elements of a pseudo-ventilation system.

Most GGVs at the cooperating site are drilled within a short distance (10–30 m (30–100 ft)) of the coalbed being mined and cased with steel pipe. Commonly, the bottom section of the casing (generally about 61 m (200 ft)) is slotted and placed adjacent to the expected gas production zone in the overburden strata. The diameter of the casing may change, but is usually around 18–20 cm (7–8 in).

Effect of Completion Parameters of Gob Gas Ventholes on Their Performance

The standard casing diameter for the GGVs in the study area was 18 cm (7 in). The effects of different slotted casing diameters (25 and 10 cm (10 and 4 in)) on methane production were evaluated. The length of the slotted casing and its setting depth above the top of the Pittsburgh Coalbed were held constant at their original design values, 61 and 12 m (200 and 40 ft), respectively.

The modeling results (Table 10) predict that the cumulative methane production using the 25-cm (10-in) casing will increase 4.9%, compared to the 18-cm (7-in) standard-diameter casing. The amount of methane produced with the 10-cm (4-in) casing was about 6.7% less than that produced with the 18-cm (7-in) diameter casing. However, the amount of mine air produced with the 10-in casing was 12% more, which resulted in a lower predicted methane concentration in the produced gas stream. The average calculated methane concentration in the produced gas stream at the end of simulated mining period (910 days) was 60% with 25-cm (10-in) casing, compared to 62% and 64% with 18- and 10-cm (7- and 4-in) diameter casing, respectively [Karacan et al. 2006].

The predicted increase in cumulative methane production with the larger-diameter wellbore was due to the increase in the open-to-flow area of the wellbore and the calculated productivity index (a mathematical means of expressing the ability of a reservoir to deliver fluids to the wellbore, stated as the volume delivered per drawdown pressure) in the wellbore models. Also, with larger-diameter wellbores, the pressure losses were less compared to smaller-diameter wellbores. The predicted reduction in methane concentration with the 25-cm (10-in) diameter casing is most likely the result of more mine air being captured due to an expanded pressure sink and associated depletion radius created by the production of gas from the larger-diameter casing. However, since the total predicted gas production (methane and air) was higher for the 25-cm (10-in) diameter casing, it still resulted in higher cumulative methane production, even though the methane concentration was less (Table 10).

Table 10.—Predicted effect of casing diameter on cumulative methane and total gas production for 910 days of simulated mining

Casing diameter, cm (in)	Cumulative methane produced, $\times 10^6$ m^3 (MMscf)	Change in methane produced compared to 7-in casing, %	Cumulative gas produced (methane + air), $\times 10^6$ m^3 (MMscf)	Change in air compared to 7-in casing, %	Calculated methane concentration, %
10 (4)	11.1 (392)	−6.7	17.3 (609)	−15	64
18 (7)	11.9 (420)	—	19.2 (677)	—	62
25.4 (10)	12.5 (440)	+4.9	20.6 (728)	+12	60

> **Increasing gob gas venthole diameter results in more methane production. However, methane concentration may be diluted due to the inclusion of more mine air. Differing coalbed reservoir parameters may modify the optimum gob gas venthole configurations.**

To evaluate the influence of the length of the completion interval on GGV performance, the length of the slotted casing section was changed in the model to 30 and 76 m (100 and 250 ft), compared to the original 61-m (200-ft) length. The casing diameter was kept at 18 cm (7 in), and the setting depth of 12 m (40 ft) above the top of the Pittsburgh Coalbed was maintained. The modeling results predict that the cumulative methane production will increase with increases in slotted casing length (Figure 23).

Methane production with 76 m (250 ft) of slotted casing was 13.0×10^6 m^3 (460 MMscf), compared to 12.1×10^6 m^3 (392 MMscf) with the standard 61 m (200 ft) of slotted casing. This difference corresponds to a 9.5% increase in methane capture from the four panels modeled (Figure 22). However, when the slotted casing length was shortened to 30 m (100 ft), the predicted methane production decreased to 8.91×10^6 m^3 (315 MMscf), which was about 25% less than that captured with 61 m (200 ft) of slotted casing.

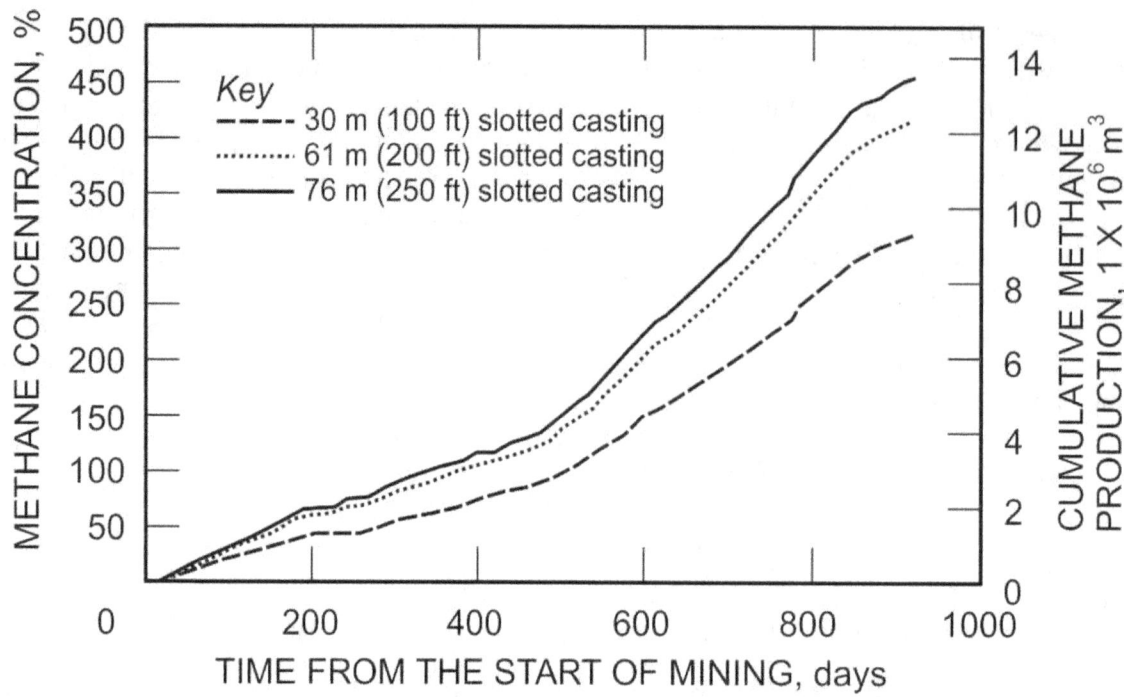

Figure 23.—Simulated cumulative methane production from ventholes with varying lengths of slotted casing.

Increasing slotted casing length results in increased methane production. Knowledge about key reservoir parameters in the overlying strata (e.g., coalbed methane content, formation permeability) can be very useful input for configuring gob gas venthole slotted casing lengths.

The effect of casing setting depth (distance from the top of the mining layer) on gas production was investigated by modeling alternative completion depths of 19.3, 7.6, and 4.6 m (65, 25, and 15 ft), compared to the original 12-m (40-ft) depth. The 7.6-m (25-ft) completion depth generally corresponded closely to the caved zone height, which was modeled as 7.3 m (24 ft) above the Pittsburgh Coalbed. Consequently, the 4.6-m (15-ft) completion depth resulted in the venthole being drilled into the caved zone. The 19.3-m (65-ft) completion depth corresponds to a depth slightly below the Sewickley Coalbed. For these scenarios, the casing diameter and slotted casing lengths were kept at their original design values, 18 cm and 61 m (7 in and 200 ft), respectively.

Raising the slotted casing setting depth to 19.8 m (65 ft), compared to 12 m (40 ft), above the Pittsburgh Coalbed resulted in a 4% predicted cumulative methane production increase. The predicted cumulative methane production declined by about 5% and 29% when the casing was set to within 7.6 and 4.6 m (25 and 15 ft) of the top of the mining layer, respectively. The total gas production increased by 4.9% with the 19.8-m (65-ft) slotted casing setting depth scenario (mostly because of the increase in methane concentration) and decreased by 5% for the 7.6-m (25-ft) setting depth (mostly because of the decrease in methane concentration). The total gas production increased by about 10% with the 4.6-m (15-ft) slotted casing setting depth. In the

4.6-m (15-ft) setting depth scenario, the lower slots of the casing were in the caved zone influenced by the mine ventilation system, where flow resistance was small. Therefore, the ventholes pulled 74% more mine air, compared to the operator's standard 12-m (40-ft) setting depth. Since most of the produced gas was mine air at the 4.6-m (15-ft) setting depth, the average methane concentration in the cumulative produced gas at the end of mining was about 40%, compared to 60%–70% average methane concentration calculated for other depths (Figure 24).

A real-world example of the gas quality consequences of completing GGVs into the caved zone is illustrated with measured gas concentration data from two ventholes continuously monitored during a field study (Figure 25). For this site, the height of the caved zone was estimated to be 12 m (40 ft). This is higher than the site shown in Figure 22 due to the presence of the sandstone paleochannel. The first venthole on the study panel was completed to a depth of 14.3 m (47 ft) above the top of the Pittsburgh Coalbed, generally within the standard depth range for the mine site. However, the second venthole drilled on the study panel was inadvertently drilled deeper to a depth of 11 m (35 ft) above the top of the Pittsburgh Coalbed, which is in the caved zone. As shown in Figure 25, the methane concentration in the produced gas from the venthole completed into the caved zone averaged about 30% less than that of the standard completion depth above the caved zone because of the increased production of mine ventilation air [Karacan et al. 2007b].

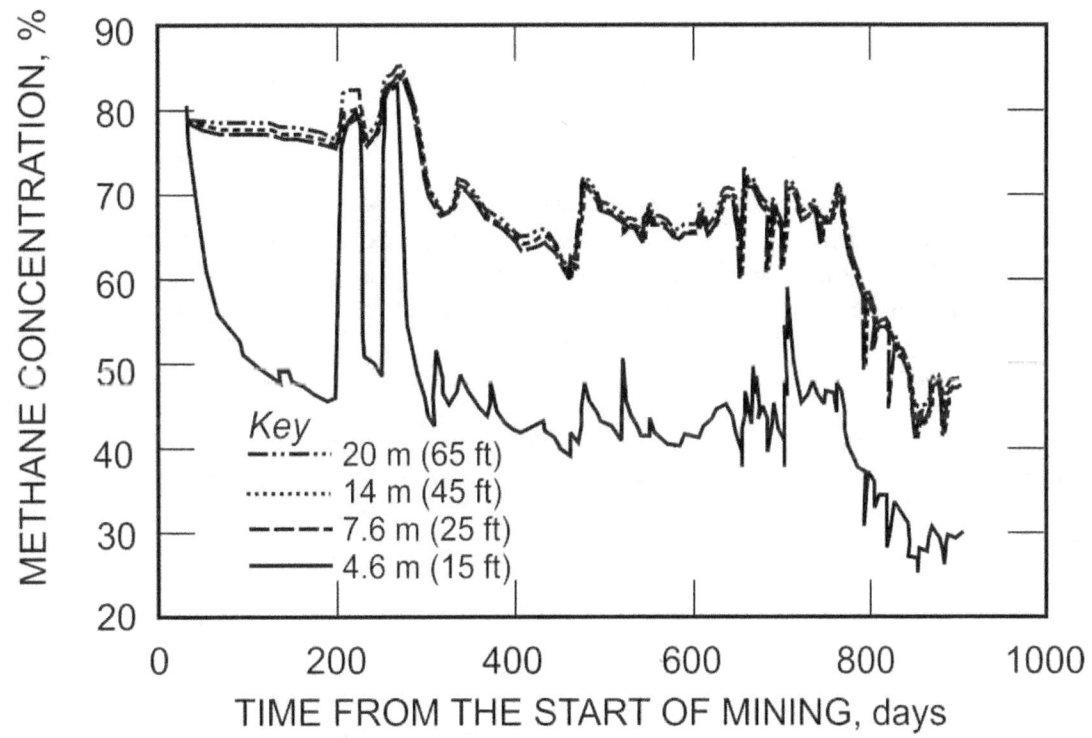

Figure 24.—Simulated methane concentrations in the gas production stream from ventholes completed to varying depths above the Pittsburgh Coalbed.

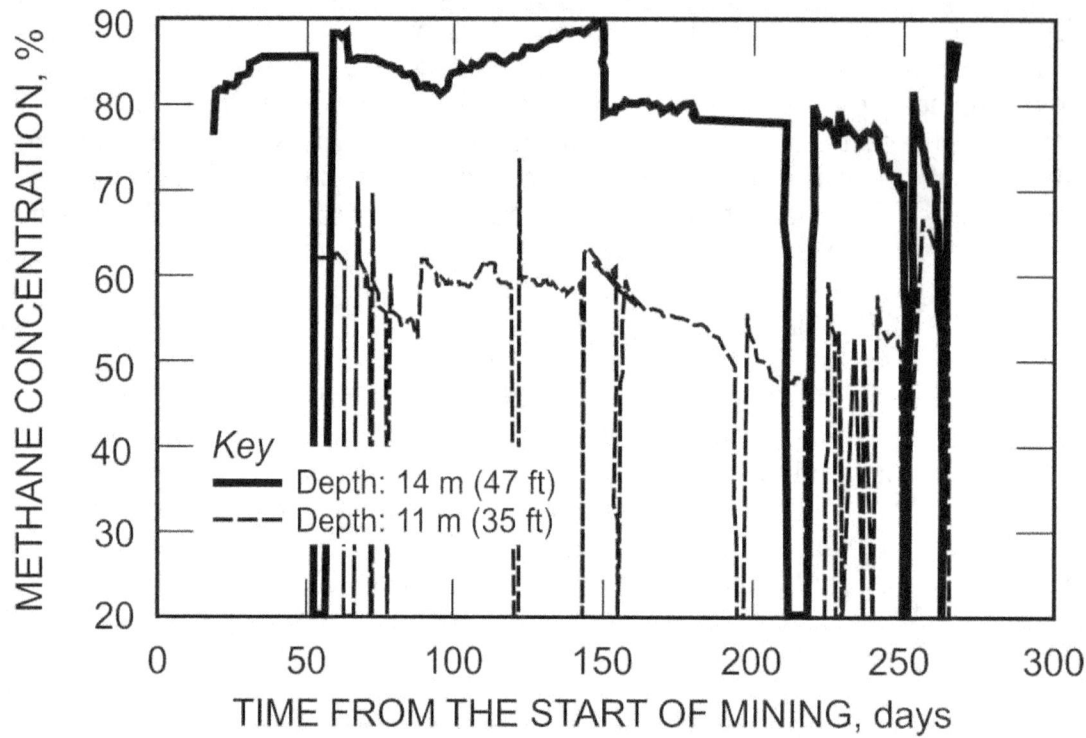

Figure 25.—Actual methane concentrations measured in the gas production stream from two GGVs completed to different depths above the Pittsburgh Coalbed on the same longwall panel.

> **Locating the bottom of gob gas ventholes into the caved zone is counterproductive for methane control because mine ventilation air is then removed from the borehole, limiting the potential removal of methane.**

The increase in mine ventilating air from the GGVs is a problem for several reasons. The first concern is that if the venthole is producing at its maximum capacity, then the borehole is producing a portion of the ventilation air and in favor of the maximum quantity of methane available in the subsided strata, which can then migrate to the underground workplace where it is a potential explosion hazard. In addition, when coalbeds and associated caved zone strata are prone to spontaneous combustion, the flow of additional mine air into this zone may pose an increased risk of a mine fire of spontaneous combustion origin [Smith et al. 1994]. There are also economic issues associated with producing higher levels of mine ventilation air from the GGVs. Obviously, there are costs associated with providing ventilation air to the underground workings, as there are with the drilling and operation of the ventholes. Economically, it is counter-productive to incur cost to first introduce the ventilation air to the mine, and then incur additional cost to remove it from the mine via the GGVs. Finally, for those mining operations capturing gob gas for commercial sale, it is very important to maintain as high a methane concentration as possible in the produced gas stream, or additional expenses will be incurred to remove the nonhydrocarbon gases prior to selling it to the pipeline.

An important factor in optimizing coalbed methane production from gob gas ventholes is surface exhauster operation. In the case of methane-powered exhausters, keeping the methane concentration high extends the production life of the gob gas venthole, since most operators will shut in boreholes when concentrations drop below 25%. Many exhauster motors powered by methane cease to run reliably when concentrations drop to levels approaching 25%, which significantly limits their effectiveness in controlling gob gas underground emissions.

Summary

- Locating the bottom of GGVs into the caved zone limits the removal of methane by using borehole capacity to remove some mine ventilation air.

- Increasing slotted casing length results in increased methane production from a GGV. Other site-specific factors need to be considered in increasing the casing length, such as the geology where the borehole will be anchored.

- Many exhauster motors powered by methane cease to run reliably when concentrations drop to levels approaching 25%, which limits their effectiveness in controlling gob gas contributions to underground emissions. Powering the surface exhauster with an alternate fuel source will allow coalbed methane production to continue without combustion performance concerns. To maintain safe operating conditions, a 25% methane concentration cutoff is commonly used for all exhauster operation.

7. THE APPLICATION OF GOB GAS VENTHOLES TO CONTROL METHANE IN WIDER LONGWALL PANELS AND GOBS

Overview

The competitive nature of the domestic and international coal industry is constantly pushing mining companies to increase coal productivity and the size of their longwall panels. Increasing panel widths can result in increased methane emissions due to the larger volumes of gas released from the surrounding and overlying strata. The design and locations of GGVs are important to control the extra amount of gas resulting from increased amount of fractured strata.

The grid model shown in Figure 26 was developed to estimate the increase in expected levels of methane emissions and to investigate alternative GGV completion and placement scenarios on a larger panel [Karacan et al. 2005]. These data were produced in a new mining district in the Pittsburgh Coalbed. Mining in the district had begun with 381-m (1,250-ft) wide panels and was progressing to 442-m (1,450-ft) wide panels.

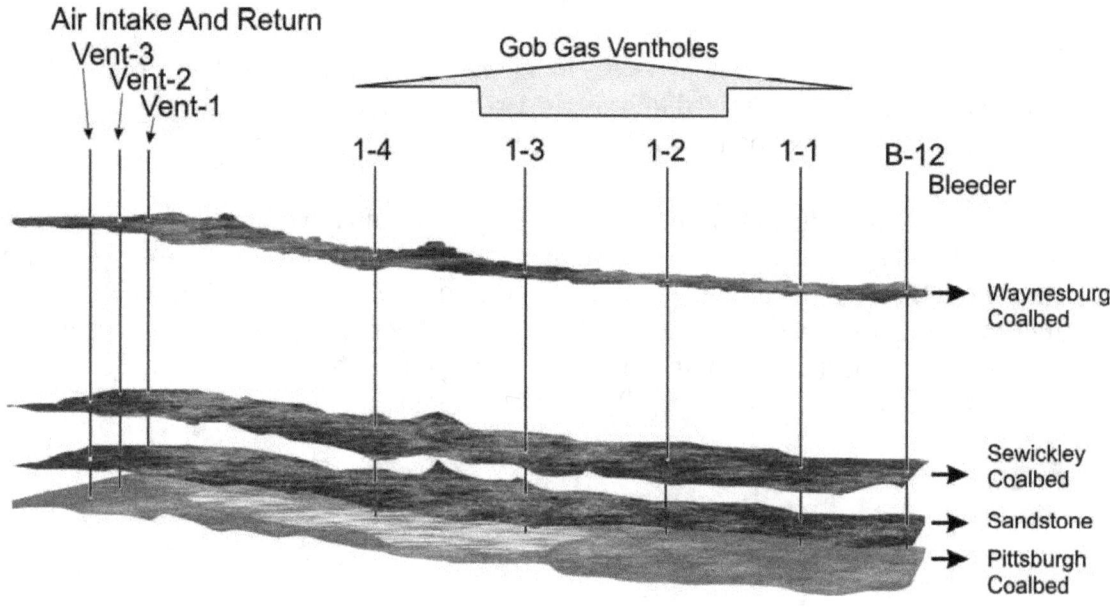

Figure 26.—Study mine for wider longwall faces: grid model of a new mining district in the Pittsburgh Coalbed.

Effects of Increased Longwall Panel Width on Gob Methane Emissions

Due to the uncertainty of the methane emission consequences associated with mining of the larger panel size, the field area was modeled to estimate the expected increase in gas flow from the gob and to investigate methane control options. The primary question to be answered from a mine safety and methane control perspective was whether the current number and configuration of GGVs would adequately control the projected increase in gob gas on the larger longwall panels [Karacan et al. 2005].

The four GGVs on the first panel in this new mining district were drilled to varying depths of 14, 11, 9, and 12 m (47, 35, 30, and 40 ft) above the top of the Pittsburgh Coalbed.

Two of the ventholes were completed into or at the top of the caved zone, as opposed to the preferred distance of at least 12 m (40 ft) above the top of the coal. The simulation results for the 381-m (1,250-ft) wide panel with the four GGVs were compared with those obtained with a panel width of 442 m (1,450 ft). The same venthole placement (91 m (300 ft) from the tailgate side of the panel) and completion and production histories were maintained (Figure 27).

The performance of the four individual GGVs on the simulated wider panel was very similar to that of the original panels. This was expected since the wellbore flow model was not dependent on panel width. Due to subsidence variations, the most likely reservoir parameter that could be influenced by increased panel width was the reservoir permeability associated with the productivity index of the ventholes. However, for supercritical panels (as are both of these simulated base cases), subsidence should be complete and stress conditions should be similar irrespective of the panel width, as confirmed by the FLAC computations [Karacan et al. 2005].

Modeling the increase in panel width resulted in 1.3×10^6 m^3 (47 MMscf) of additional methane liberation from the coal mined on the longwall face and 3.88×10^6 m^3 (137 MMscf) from the overlying disturbed strata, for a total of 5.21×10^6 m^3 (184 MMscf) of additional methane over the 268 days of mining simulated for this study. The 1.3×10^6 m^3 (47 MMscf) of additional methane liberation on the face will flow to the ventilation system unless it is predrained from the mined coalbed. Alternatively, the ventilation airflow may have to be increased to dilute the additional gas. Depending on the availability of additional gob gas drainage capacity, some of the additional 3.88×10^6 m^3 (137 MMscf) of methane originating in the overlying strata may flow to the ventilation system. This would represent the potential of up to about 0.168 m^3/s (355 cfm) of additional methane entering the underground workplace.

> **Increasing the longwall panel width increases the quantity of methane present due to the increased fractured reservoir volume. However, this size increase does not positively affect the performance of GGVs. Thus, to avoid additional methane emissions to the ventilation system associated with increased panel size, an optimized methane control system may be required.**

Comparison of Ideally Completed and Operated Gob Gas Boreholes With Those Operating in the Field

Simulations were conducted to replace the four simulated actual ventholes with four optimal[5] ventholes on the 442-m (1,450-ft) wide panel. As shown in Figure 28, optimal ventholes produced gas that was 85%–90% methane during the entire mining period, whereas the methane concentration of the gas produced by the actual wells in the study area declined significantly with time, with the methane concentration in the 65%–70% range for most of the mining period. The difference in methane concentrations between the two scenarios is due to the fact that some of the actual ventholes were drilled into or very close to the caved zone; thus, their produced methane was diluted with mine ventilation air.

---

[5]Regularly maintained and continuously operated.

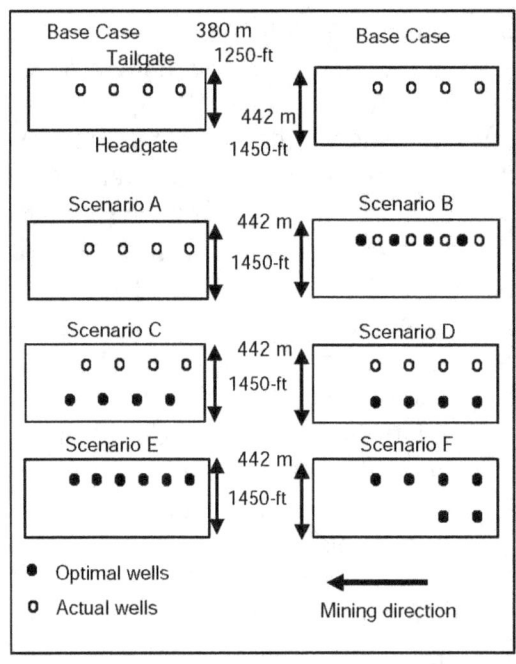

Figure 27.—Schematic representation of GGV configurations for the simulation of methane control options on wider longwall panels.

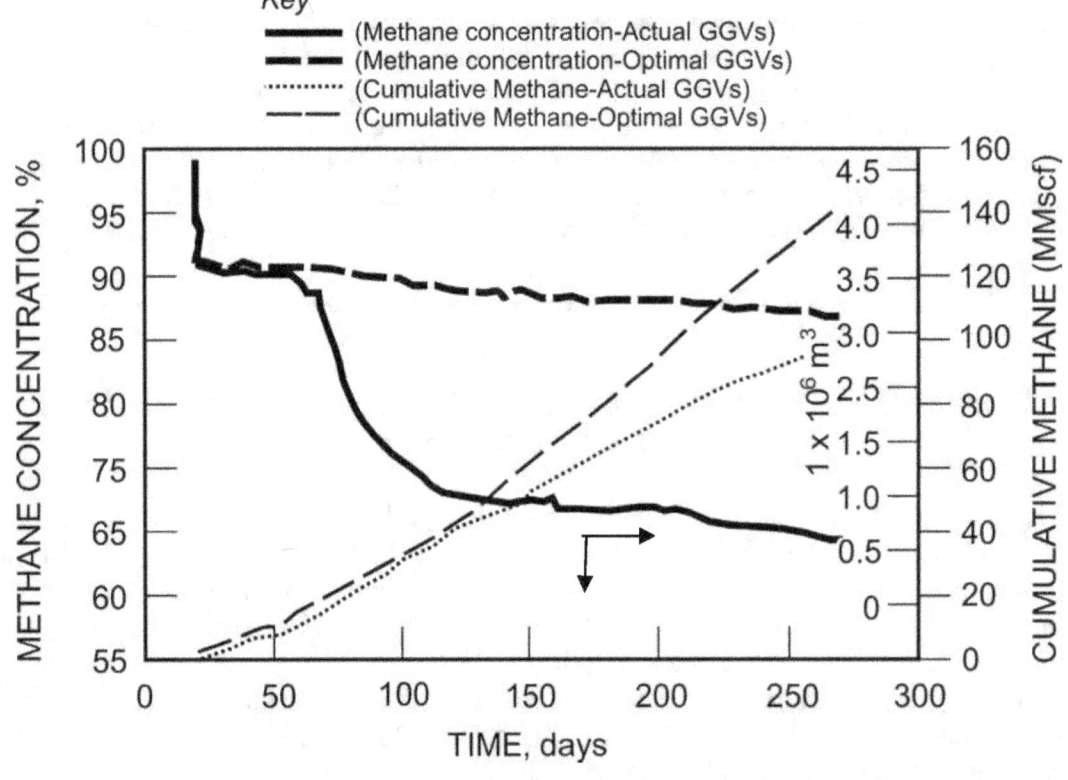

Figure 28.—Comparison of the performance of actual GGVs at the study site with the optimal GGVs for the 442-m (1,450-ft) wide panel.

Optimal wells were also predicted to produce about 50% more methane than the actual wells. This, again, demonstrates the importance of implementing proper venthole completion practices and paying close attention to the maintenance and operation of the GGVs, i.e., keeping them running to optimize their methane control capability.

> **Optimally drilled and continuously operated GGVs produced more methane at higher concentrations compared to their counterparts that were diluted by ventilation air and operated discontinuously. Although some operators prefer to keep GGV completion depths near the mined coalbed, these operators risk short-lived and intermittent GGV production.**

Since the performance (gas production potential) of individual GGVs was not influenced significantly by an increased panel width, the additional 0.168 m^3/s (355 cfm) of methane released from the overlying strata as a result of mining the larger panel will potentially enter the underground workplace if additional methane drainage capacity is not provided. Thus, the constructed model was used to evaluate multiple scenarios to optimize the number and locations of the GGVs on the wider panel and to minimize the volume of additional methane entering the ventilation system.

The simulated alternative GGV placement and completion scenarios investigated for this study, as shown in Figure 27, were: (A) moving the four actual ventholes to locations 152 m (500 ft) from tailgate side, i.e., 61 m (200 ft) closer to the centerline of the panel than on the first panel; (B) adding four optimal boreholes continuously operating with 19-kPa (2.7-psi) suction pressure and completed to 12 m (40 ft) above the Pittsburgh Coalbed located between each actual venthole; (C) adding four optimal ventholes located 91 m (300 ft) from the gate roads on the headgate side of the panel and positioned diagonally to the actual ventholes; and (D) adding four optimal ventholes located 91 m (300 ft) from the gate roads on the headgate side and positioned directly opposite the actual ventholes on the tailgate. Also, two scenarios with all optimal ventholes were tested (E and F) for their production performance and for reducing methane emissions into the ventilation system.

The data presented in Table 11 compare the cumulative methane production volumes from each of the GGV configuration scenarios shown in Figure 27. The lowest predicted cumulative methane production (scenario A) is obtained when the four ventholes with the actual completions are located 152 m (500 ft) from the tailgate entry of the 442-m (1,450-ft) panel. This configuration produced 0.37 × 10^6 m^3 (13 MMscf) less methane compared to the base case production from the 381-m (1,250-ft) panel, where the ventholes were the traditional 91 m (300 ft) from the gate road, which illustrates the importance of near-margin venthole placement [Diamond et al. 1994].

The highest predicted cumulative methane production is achieved when additional optimal ventholes are used (Table 11). To demonstrate, scenario D produces 3.91 × 10^6 m^3 (138 MMscf) more methane compared to the four actual ventholes on the 3,810-m (1,250-ft) panel base case. Scenario C was the next highest incremental producer of methane at 3.37 × 10^6 m^3 (119 MMscf). Although scenarios C and D are similar, scenario D is probably the higher producer because the tailgate and headgate ventholes are closer to each other (since they are directly opposite each other on the panel) and are intercepted by mining at the same time. This scenario results in a quicker overlap of the venthole drainage radii, which enhances gas desorption from the overlying coalbeds associated with the subsided strata. Also, when headgate and tailgate ventholes are intercepted at the same time, the headgate ventholes start producing earlier and stay on production longer compared to the diagonal location in scenario C, which results in more methane production. Within the scenarios evaluated, the third highest incremental methane producer is scenario B, with 3.19×10^6 m^3 (113 MMscf) more methane than the four actual ventholes on the 381-m (1,250-ft) panel.

The application of GGVs located on the headgate site of a longwall panel may seem counterintuitive to many seasoned methane control experts who have traditionally used the tailgate side of the panel. Other than the numerical modeling result, there are other supporting lines of evidence for this approach. Tracer gas testing performed by the NIOSH Pittsburgh Research Laboratory (PRL) in longwall gobs showed very long-ranged effects of a GGV over the length of a longwall panel. By splitting GGV locations between the headgate and tailgate near-margin locations, fewer boreholes are competing for gas in the fractured overburden, enhancing production potential. Tailgate locations are always the preferred site for cross-measure boreholes where the underground ventilation system assists in transporting methane-air mixtures through the mining-induced fracture system. For headgate-side GGVs to be effective, they must be completed above the caved zone, and induced mine fractures must not extend to ventilation pathways. The first report of the near-margin GGV design produced by the USBM used holes on the headgate side of a longwall panel due to land accessibility restrictions and achieved favorable results [Diamond et al. 1994].

One of the main considerations in GGV design and operation is to locate and drill the ventholes optimally and operate them continuously. This will minimize the number of ventholes that need to be drilled to produce the same amount of methane that a larger number of less than optimally drilled and operated ventholes will produce. Thus, in addition to the GGV placement scenarios (A through D), scenarios E and F were simulated to determine the minimum number of optimal ventholes that would produce the same maximum amount of methane as in the highest-producer configuration of actual and optimal ventholes. In scenario E, six optimal ventholes were placed along the tailgate side of the panel. In scenario F, two of the optimal ventholes were placed on the headgate side directly opposite the first two ventholes on the tailgate side.

Table 11.—Cumulative predicted methane production difference
from gob gas ventholes on a 442-m (1,450-ft) wide panel

Venthole design	Cumulative methane production difference compared to a 381-m (1,250-ft) wide face, $\times 10^3$ m^3 (MMscf)
442-m (1,450-ft)	−25
Base case	−0.9
Scenario A	−370 (−13)
Scenario B	3,200 (113)
Scenario C	3,370 (119)
Scenario D	3,910 (138)
Scenario E	2,440 (86)
Scenario F	3,790 (134)

The predicted methane production performance of venthole configurations in scenarios E and F using six optimal GGVs were compared to the performance of scenario D, the highest predicted methane producer (3.91×10^6 m^3 (138 MMscf)) in the previous simulations. Table 11 shows that scenario E, where six optimal ventholes were located along the tailgate side of the panel, produced about 2.44×10^6 m^3 (86 MMscf) more methane than the 381-m (1,250-ft) base case, whereas scenario F, with two of the optimal wells on the headgate side, produced 3.79×10^6 m^3 (134 MMscf) more methane. Thus, the six optimal ventholes of scenario F produced almost as much methane as the eight (four actual and four optimal) ventholes of scenario D. The predicted performance differences between scenarios E and F are due to the location of the ventholes and the length of time they stayed on production.

Analyses show that six optimally completed, placed, and operated ventholes could produce the same amount of methane on the wider panel as eight nonoptimal wells. Increasing the production of gob gas decreases the methane emissions into the mining environment by reducing the amount of gas unremoved by methane drainage.

Summary

- Increasing the longwall panel width increases the quantity of methane present in the gob, but does not positively affect the flow and methane concentration produced from GGVs.

- To avoid additional methane emissions to the ventilation system associated with increased panel size, an optimized methane control system may be required.

- Optimally drilled GGVs produced more methane at higher concentrations compared to ventholes that were diluted by ventilation air.

- When completing GGVs to depths near the mined coalbed, operators risk short-lived and intermittent venthole production.

- Six optimally completed, placed, and operated ventholes can produce the same amount of methane on the wider panel as eight nonoptimal wells.

8. INDUCED FRACTURING AND COALBED GAS MIGRATION IN LONGWALL PANEL OVERBURDEN: THE NIOSH BOREHOLE MONITORING EXPERIMENT

Overview

The predictive capability of numerical models can be improved by a better understanding of underground processes using site-specific field measurement data. To better understand the longwall mining effects on the methane reservoir overlying a longwall panel and to provide data for ongoing PRL modeling efforts, a borehole monitoring experiment (BME) was designed and implemented on an active longwall panel. The mine operates in the Pittsburgh Coalbed in Greene County, Pennsylvania. The goal of the BME is to provide recommendations to operators related to improving methane control measures through field observations of this study and through field-monitoring-assisted reservoir modeling technique enhancements. This section discusses the BME and the most important measurements, results, and recommendations associated with this effort.

Description of the Borehole Monitoring Experiment on an Active Longwall Panel

The boreholes were drilled in a new mining district where a prior longwall panel had been previously described by numerical models. The BME provides a direct comparison of field site observations to previous numerical experiments and also allows construction of refined models of the mined area for more accurate and detailed analysis. The drill site was selected based on an active panel, and all borehole activity was completed (except for monitoring) prior to undermining by the longwall face. The BME site location was chosen to be away from either end of the panel to avoid mechanical influences caused by the draping of overburden in this region. The borehole drilling depths and monitoring intervals were initially chosen to address a different stratigraphic zone in each hole. The experimental design specified that drilling was to be completed 2 months in advance of undermining the borehole location.

The BME was planned for a panel that was 442 m (1,450 ft) wide. The three test boreholes were arranged in a line that was equidistant from the tailgate gate roads. The distance to the tailgate panel margin was 101 m (330 ft), the same distance that the mine used for its GGVs so that they would be in the same mechanical behavior zone and in a similar stress field. One of the operator's GGVs was to be drilled 1,930 m (6,325 ft) from the completion end of the panel and was to be included in the BME monitoring activities. The distances between each of the monitoring boreholes was 15 m (50 ft), and the third borehole was 76 m (250 ft) from the nearby GGV.

The three test boreholes were drilled and completed at different depths to monitor initial reservoir and mechanical properties in different strata horizons and subsequent property changes during the mining of the longwall panel. The top of the Pittsburgh Coalbed was at 252 m (827 ft) from the surface. According to this plan, the first, or shallowest, borehole (BH–1) was drilled to a total depth of 220 m (721 ft). The second, or midrange borehole (BH–2), was drilled to a depth of 230 m (755 ft). The deepest borehole (BH–3), which was also closest to the GGV, was drilled to 245 m (803 ft).

Based on the local geology and the depths of the boreholes shown in Figure 29, BH–1 was intended to monitor the Sewickley Coalbed, BH–2 to monitor mostly shale sequences, and

BH–3 (the deepest) to monitor the shale and sandstone horizons that would be retained in the gob during and after undermining. Boreholes were drilled with a 15-cm (6-in) diameter bit. The drilling of the boreholes was started and completed when the longwall face was 760 m (2,500 ft) away from the BH–1 location. After drilling was completed, the deepest borehole (BH–3) was logged open-hole with density, gamma ray, and sonic tools to identify the formations, refine the drilling depths, and calculate porosity, density, and some of the mechanical properties of the rock.

The boreholes were cased with 13-cm (5-in) steel casing. They were cemented using conventional grout and cement baskets, except for the bottom 6.1–9.1 m (20–30 ft). These sections were cased with slotted casing and were the primary monitoring zones for each hole. The length of slotted casing was 9.1 m (30 ft) in BH–1 in order to monitor both splits of the Sewickley Coalbed. The last 2.4 m (8 ft) of the slotted casing of BH–3 was cut and left open-hole to keep the casing as high as possible above the gob (Figure 29).

The experimental boreholes were configured to be completed in a manner similar to the mine operator's GGVs. Both borehole designs include flame arrestors, shut-in valves, and a long, vertical PVC pipe stack. However, unlike the experimental boreholes, the GGVs were cased with 61-m (200-ft) slotted casing at the bottom of all boreholes. The operator used a dump grouting procedure on the GGVs instead of the circulating grout method used on the test boreholes. The test boreholes were also different from the operator's GGVs in that the BME boreholes were kept shut in throughout the mining duration and a powered exhauster was not attached.

After the cementing operation, all of the boreholes were blown dry of any water remaining after completing the cementing operation by tripping the drill tubing down into the boreholes and using compressed air from the drill rig. Similar to the GGVs, test borehole wellheads were equipped with 15-cm (6-in) diameter flange for installation of the flame arrestor and the wellhead valve. Borehole monitoring instrumentation and associated hardware were also attached to the borehole stack.

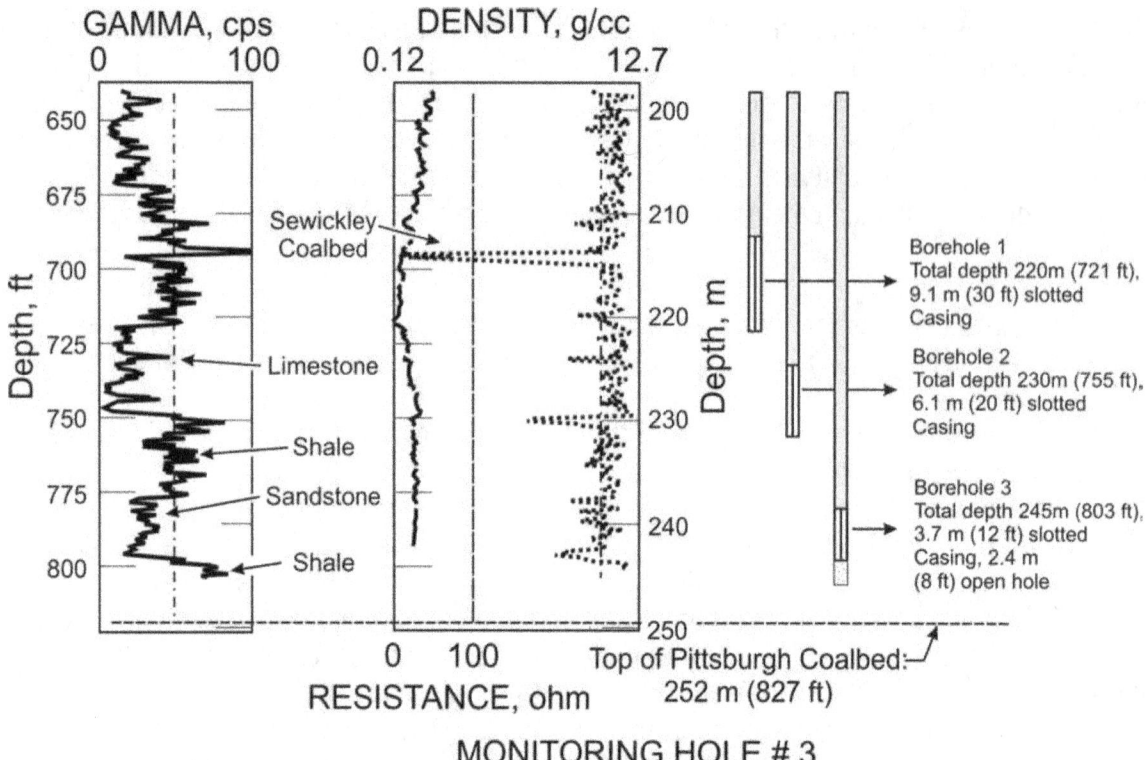

Figure 29.—Stratigraphy and downhole configurations for NIOSH BME. (TD = total depth.)

Methodology and Instrumentation

An important part of this study was to perform measurements of in situ permeability before and after the undermining of the NIOSH drill sites. To make these measurements, an experimental method was designed. These tests also provided valuable data on water production from the slotted casing sections. The initial, pre-undermining findings present data on the initial water saturations of the formations of interest. Initial permeability determinations were first conducted by using a rising-head test before installing the wellheads and shutting in the wells for long-term monitoring.

For this test, boreholes were equipped with submersible, downhole transducers that were positioned within the downhole monitoring zones. The downhole transducers were to be installed underwater in the boreholes to record transient changes of the water head in the boreholes. However, there was no water rise recorded within a few days of borehole monitoring. Thus, a set of slug tests was designed and performed in each borehole using water to determine formation permeabilities. The water head drop was monitored for about a week on each borehole using the submersible, downhole transducers until the rate of water head change reached a steady state. After the conclusion of the initial slug tests, the downhole pressure transducers were repositioned just above the slotted sections.

The boreholes were then filled with additional quantities of water so that the change in water head could be observed. This water monitoring interval was included to provide input on strata disturbances, their initiation with respect to the position of the longwall face, and the transient fracture permeabilities induced by mining. The submersible transducers recorded changes of water head until the water drained completely from the boreholes. A final set of slug tests was to be run after the completion of the panel for determining final permeabilities.

In addition to submersible transducers, the wellheads on BME boreholes were equipped with surface pressure transducers for continuous data-recording pressure changes at the tops of the boreholes. Tiltmeters were also installed on the BME wellhead stacks for recording subsidence and strata response profiles. Conventional positional surveys were scheduled to track the movement of the surface. The longwall face position was recorded daily. Surface pressure and methane concentration readings were taken regularly to monitor the changes in the wellbores as a result of fracturing of strata. Pressure, flow rate, and concentration readings were also monitored at the nearby GGV to evaluate the underground interactions with the NIOSH boreholes. Figure 30 shows the wellhead configuration of one of the experimental boreholes.

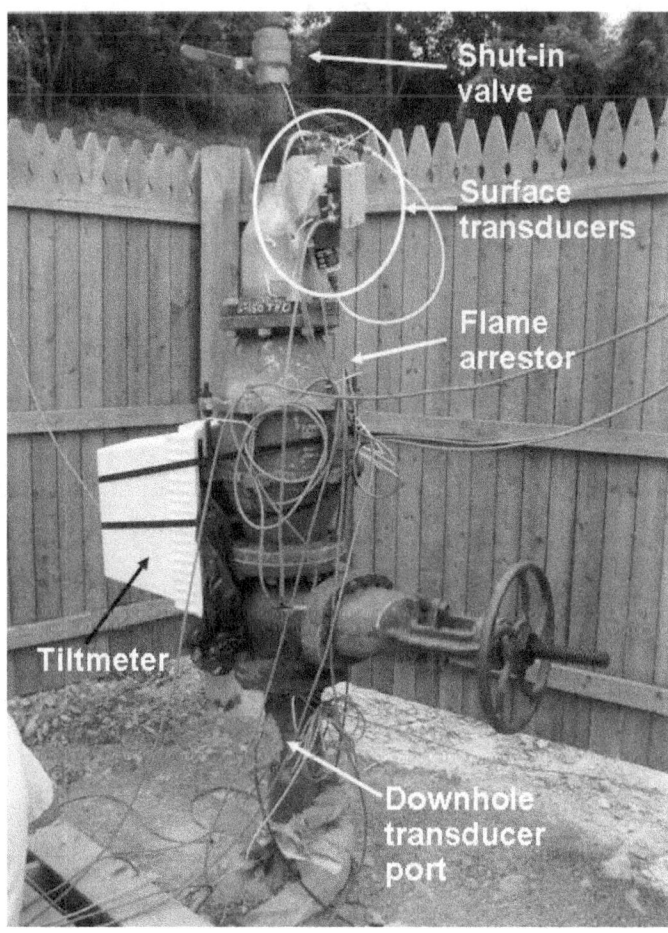

Figure 30.—Wellhead arrangement for monitoring boreholes.

A distance of 305 m (1,000 ft) before and after the NIOSH boreholes were undermined was selected as the primary experiment test zone. This distance was based on the overburden depth and typical subsidence profiles from the Northern Appalachian Basin. All instrumentation was installed, the boreholes were shut in, and monitoring had begun while the longwall face was 366 m (1,200 ft) away from the first borehole.

Analysis and Interpretation of the Field Data

Figure 31 shows the change in water head pressure in the first borehole (Sewickley Coalbed) and second borehole (shale and limestone zone between the Pittsburgh and Sewickley Coalbeds). Unfortunately, soon after starting to record data from the deepest borehole (Pittsburgh Coalbed), the communication with the downhole pressure transducer was lost. Thus, Figure 31 does not include data from the third borehole. Figure 31 shows the effect of mining disturbances on water level changes in the boreholes. The data show that the initial water head drop in the first and second boreholes occurred before the boreholes were undermined. This suggests that the initial water head decrease is associated with fracturing and/or shearing of the strata ahead of the face by about 3 days in BH–1 and about 2 days in BH–2.

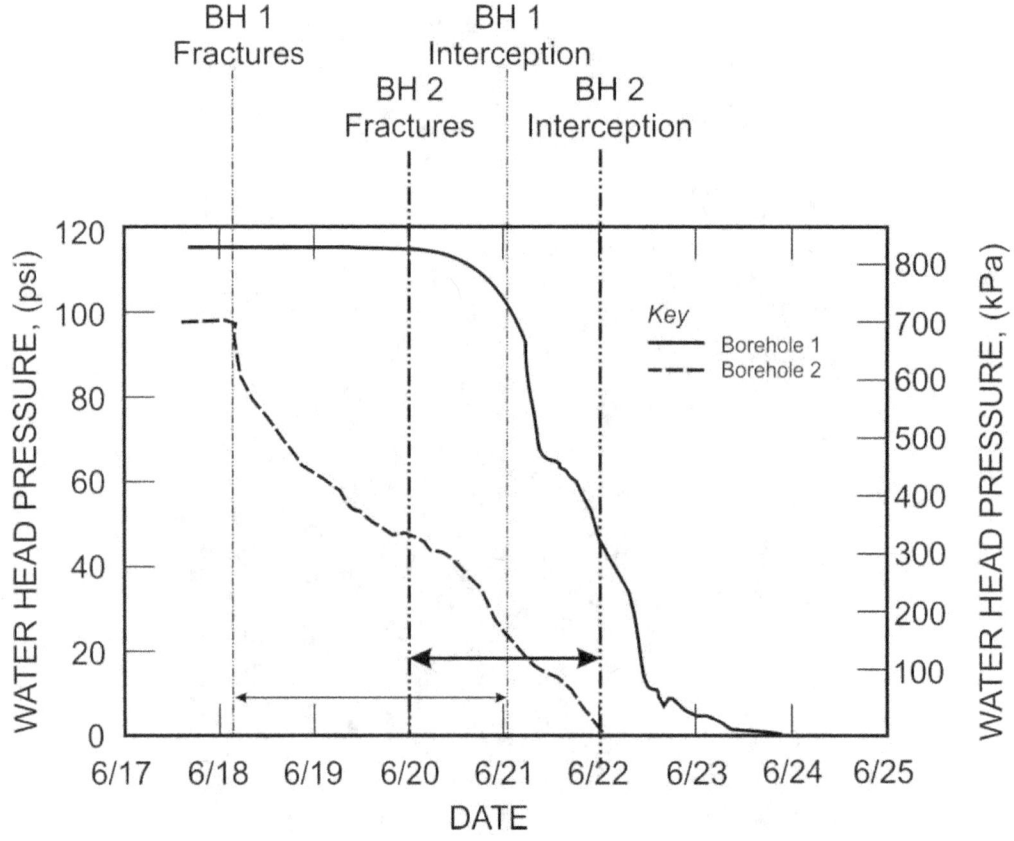

Figure 31.—Water head change as a function of time in boreholes monitoring Sewickley (BH–1) and shale-limestone (BH–2) intervals.

Figure 31 has other implications with regard to impacts of longwall mining on reservoir properties. For instance, the water level drop confirms that there are new permeability pathways created either by the shearing or by fracturing of strata. Also, the changing rate of water head drop confirms that permeability is not constant and varies (increases and decreases) as strata respond to changing stress conditions during mining.

> **Water head drop data suggest that mining-induced disturbances forming the GGV fracture network can occur 24–46 m (80–150 ft) ahead of the mining face. This distance may vary when GGV slotted pipe configurations are used, which are typically 5–10 times longer than those used in the BME.**

The data obtained during initial slug tests were evaluated by using the confined aquifer slug test model presented by Dawson and Istok [1991]. The calculated permeabilities for the monitoring zones in BH–1, BH–2, and BH–3 were 2.8, 0.1, and 0.2 md for the Sewickley Coalbed, for shale and limestone, and for shales, respectively. These evaluations also showed that these values are very close to the initial permeability values being used by NIOSH researchers in the numerical reservoir and fracture mechanics modeling these formations.

> **In monitoring water levels in the boreholes, the loss of water can be rapid up to about 32 m (100 ft) above the mined coalbed, which can limit the duration of monitoring. The rate of water loss was not related to the depth of the borehole. Shearing and deformation in the overburden is typically severe, and much of the annulus is generally modified.**

To quantify permeability changes in the overlying strata during mining, a slug test model for confined, anisotropic aquifers of infinite or semi-infinite in radial extent was used [Dawson and Istok 1991]. The model was used for calculating instantaneous permeabilities that are represented by two consecutive data points recorded in 1-min intervals and also for calculating the average permeabilities during intervals that can be recognized by abrupt changes in the rate of water head drop. Figure 32 shows the calculated permeabilities for the changes in the Sewickley Coalbed in BH–1. Figure 32A is a plot of calculated instantaneous permeabilities, while Figure 32B shows a running average of the same data.

The data show that as soon as the strata are affected by mining disturbances, the permeability increases and water head starts to drop suddenly. The value of this initial permeability increase is 700 md. After this initial increase, permeability decreases to about 100-md levels. This permeability change may indicate that initial reservoir disturbance is due to strata or bedding plane shear and fracturing, where permeability initially increases during initial movements of the strata. The permeabilities drop to a lower and uniform value (~100 md) after that. This permeability persists until about a half-day before the borehole location is undermined by the longwall face, which causes permeability to increase mostly due to shearing, horizontal fracturing, and vertical fracturing. After the borehole is undermined, permeability increases to larger values (>1,000 md) due to larger-scale fractures.

Figure 32B shows water head change and permeability evolution averaged in some distinctive segments during mining for BH–1. This figure also shows that the highest permeabilities measured in the borehole occur just after disturbances first affect the coalbed, during initial ground movement, and during undermining of the borehole location. The average fracture permeability in the Sewickley horizon during this time interval was calculated as 540 md.

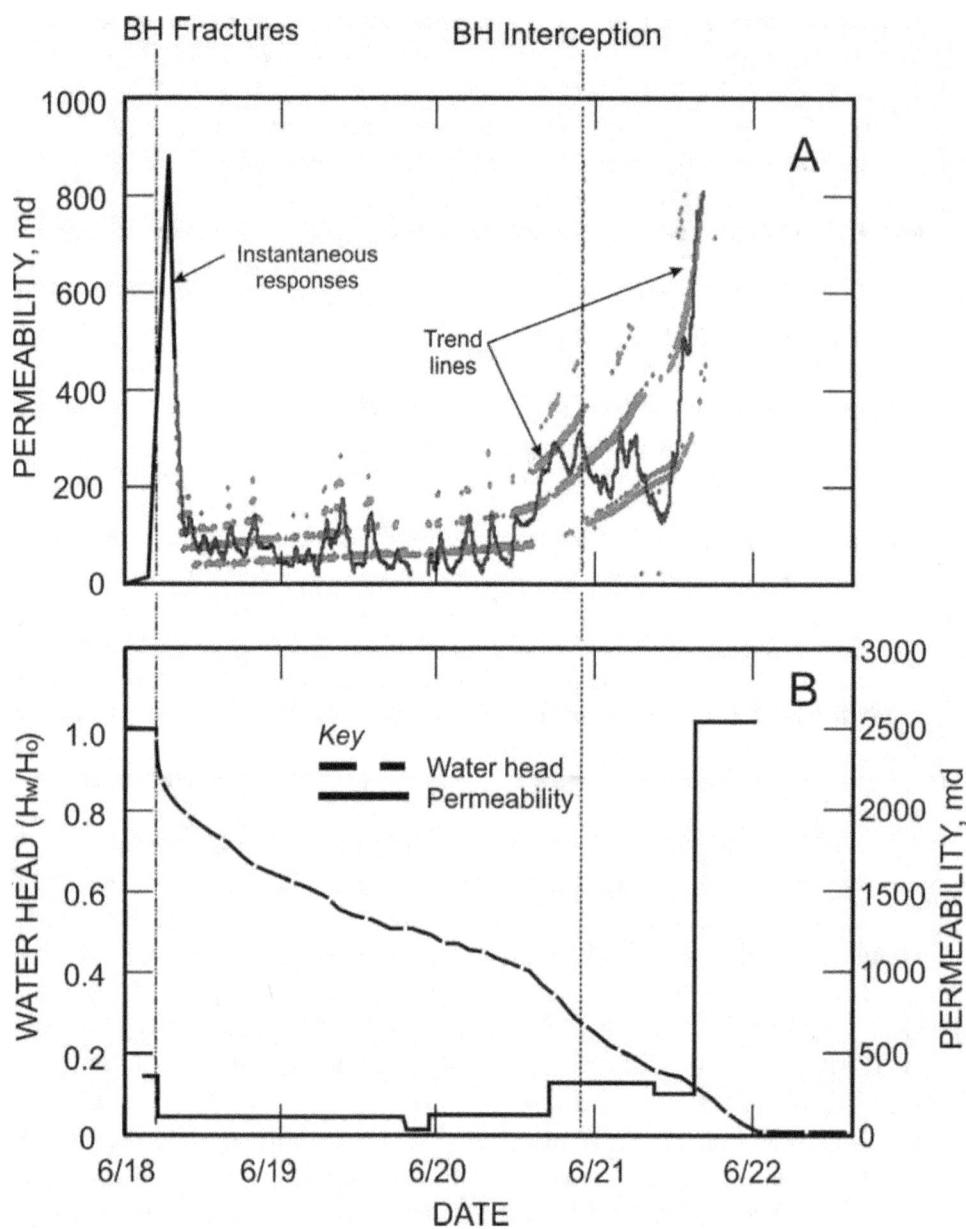

Figure 32.—A: BH-1 instantaneous change in the permeabilities of monitored horizons during mining; B: BH-1 average permeabilities at certain intervals of water head drop during mining. (H_w = height of water; H_o = initial height of water.)

BH-2, designed to monitor a 6.1-m (20-ft) section in the shale and limestone zone between the Sewickley and Pittsburgh Coalbeds, was analyzed using the same model. Figures 33A and 33B present the instantaneous and average permeabilities, respectively, within different segments identified based on the changes in the rate of water head drop for BH-2. Although this borehole is deeper and closer to mining than BH-1, this interval does not show the sudden water head loss as observed in the first borehole when mining influence reached the borehole location. Instead, the change in the water level is more gradual. This may be due to the combination of different structural and mechanical properties of this horizon compared to the BH-1 test horizon, which included the Sewickley Coalbed.

72

The data in Figure 33A show that permeabilities in BH–2 gradually increase to the 100–200 md range, possibly because of bedding plane movements. A sudden drop in water head follows this period with an associated permeability increase to about 600 md. This increase coincides with the approach of the longwall face (15 m (50 ft) away) and may suggest communication between these two wells. After this permeability increase, the values begin to decrease to the 200–300 md range, followed by a gradual increase. The permeability increases coincide with the longwall face approach until the borehole location is undermined. After undermining, large-scale horizontal and vertical fractures are created, and the permeability increases to about >1,000–1,500 md.

> **Permeabilities measured prior to undermining were in the ~1-md range. Permeability increases following undermining were dramatic, with increases of about 100–500 times and instantaneous increases of up to about 1,000 times.**

Figure 33B shows the same observations for BH–2 by presenting the average permeabilities in various segments during water head drop. This figure also shows that permeability starts increasing gradually as the mining face advances toward the borehole location until it is undermined, after which the permeabilities increase suddenly. This behavior suggests that before undermining, the fractures in the formation develop gradually. The average fracture permeability in this zone during mining was calculated as 560 md.

> **Formation permeabilities gradually increase as mining-induced disturbances progress to the borehole locations. However, the biggest change occurs with the interception of borehole locations.**

Surface Measurements of Borehole Gas

The change in methane concentrations and static pressures in the boreholes were monitored at the surface after the boreholes were shut in. These concentration and pressure measurements are shown in Figures 34A and 34B, respectively. As of July 2006, all three boreholes were intercepted during the week just before the miner's vacation, when the longwall did not operate. The GGV was intercepted after longwall mining resumed. The coal production stoppage associated with the miner's vacation and the date when the nearest GGV began gob gas production are also indicated in Figure 33.

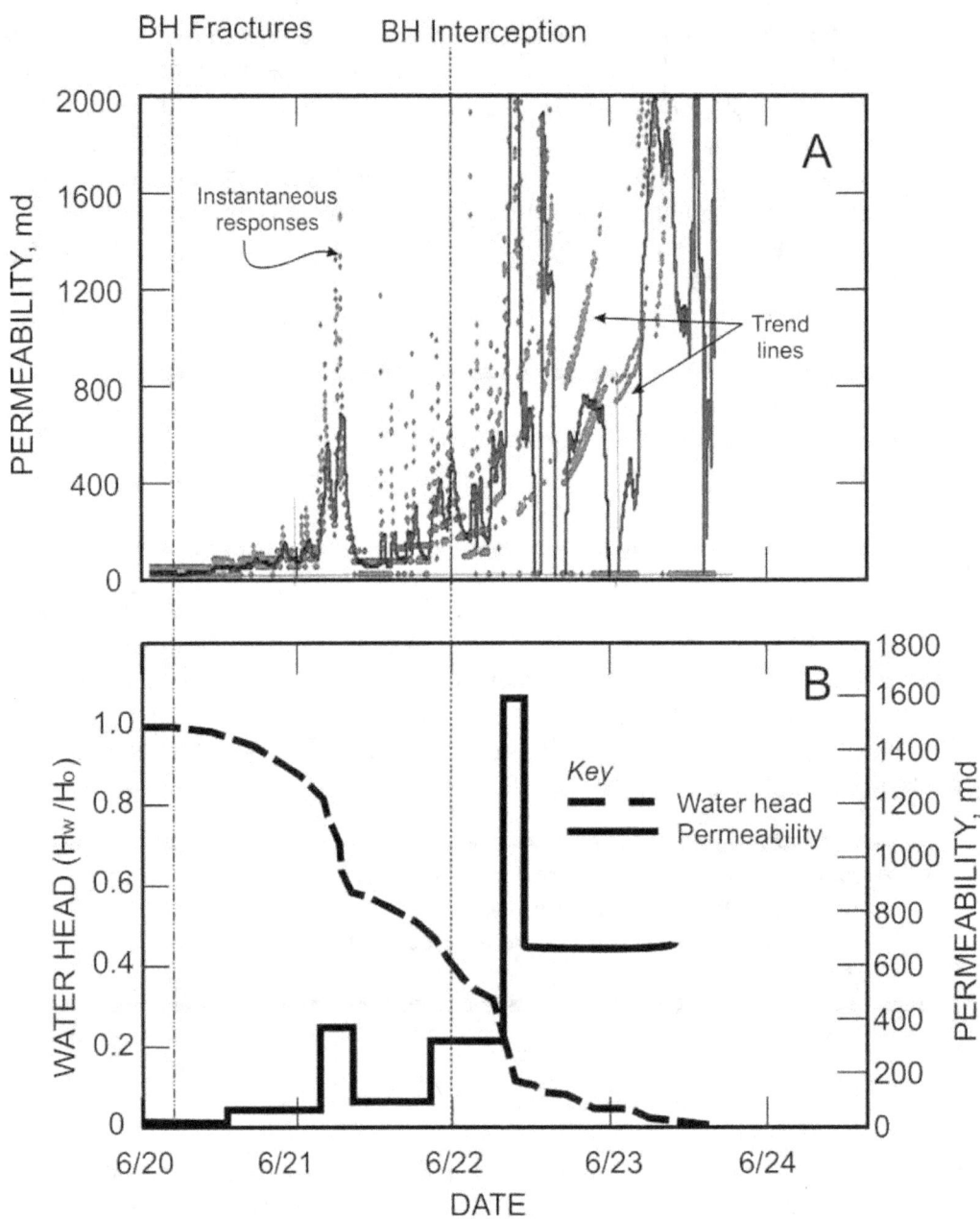

Figure 33.—A: BH–2 instantaneous change in the permeabilities of monitored horizons during mining; B: BH–2 average permeabilities. (H_w = height of water; H_o = initial height of water.)

The monitoring of downhole underwater pressures began before mining disturbances reached the borehole locations. This period is characterized by almost constant methane levels and static borehole pressures (BH–1) until the mining-related disturbances reach the borehole locations. The data show that until shearing occurred, which resulted in an initial water head drop, methane concentration was around 75%, which is the initial reading shown. Gas concentration then increased to about 85% within a few days and pressure increased to 20 cm (8 in) of water gauge in the borehole. These increases suggest that the coalbed was producing methane that was migrating into the borehole. However, when mining disturbances reached the BH–1 borehole location, concentration decreased to 40% and pressure dropped to 10 cm (4 in) of water gauge until interception (shaded portion in Figure 34), which resulted in a further decrease. However, after this borehole location was intercepted by the longwall face and all the water was drained out, methane concentration started to increase to 90%–100% because of fracturing of the coalbed and the absence of water in the boreholes.

The interception of BH–2, which monitored shale and limestone layers, showed a different behavior. Initial methane readings in this borehole before undermining were around 10% and the shut-in pressures were low, indicating that there was not significant methane flow into the borehole, probably due to low permeabilities and the presence of water in the borehole. However, after it was undermined and the water drained out, methane concentration increased to 90%–100% in the borehole with a sudden pressure fluctuation. This is possibly due to development of horizontal and vertical fractures and the associated permeability increase in the monitoring zone. The loss of water from the boreholes into mining-induced fractures following undermining resulted in the end of meaningful transducer pressure measurements and therefore the termination of the downhole permeability data.

It is also interesting to note the similar behavior of methane concentration change in BH–1 and BH–2 after undermining. This behavior suggests that these two boreholes monitored two different horizons that were about 11 m (35 ft) away from each other, and they started to communicate through horizontal and vertical fractures. This observation shows that the layers within 24 m (80 ft) of the top of the coalbed being mined are either fractured or there is enough shearing or opening of natural fractures that the formations can interact with each other. However, the fact that the mine ventilation pressures (−8 to −10 cm (−3 to −4 in) water gauge) have not been continuously recorded at these elevations suggests that there was either no direct communication with the mine or that the positive gas pressure into the boreholes from the monitored zones was high enough to compensate the negative pressure influence of mine ventilation.

The behavior of pressure and concentration data produced by BH–3, an interval about 6.1 m (20 ft) above the Pittsburgh Coalbed, is completely different from that of the other two boreholes. In BH–3, the decrease of methane concentration and shut-in pressure after mining showed that this borehole started to communicate with the mine atmosphere. After undermining, the shut-in pressure decreased to mine ventilation pressures and stayed as such for the rest of the monitoring. Also, methane concentrations decreased to very low values from 35%–45% levels before undermining. After undermining, concentration began slowly increasing to about 5% methane. Then the GGV exhauster, 76 m (250 ft) away, began to operate with a high flow rate following undermining. This resulted in an initial decrease in borehole methane concentration followed by a concentration rise in the gob, as recorded in BH–3.

The start of the nearby GGV operation is also noticeable in the other two BME boreholes (Figure 34). Although this venthole did not operate continuously and successfully because of mechanical problems after an initially high production rate, the data confirm that the venthole was communicating with the monitoring boreholes through fractures and bedding plane separations, as previously observed by Mucho et al. [2000]. The methane concentration increase in the gob (or in BH–3) may be due to an increase in methane height in the gob as a result of the negative pressure generated by the venthole blower. This rise may also be due to drawing gas from other horizons into a more permeable gob following undermining. This may also explain the decrease in BH–1 and BH–2 shut-in pressures and the decrease in measured methane concentrations associated with a concentration increase in BH–3, before the recovery again to 70% methane.

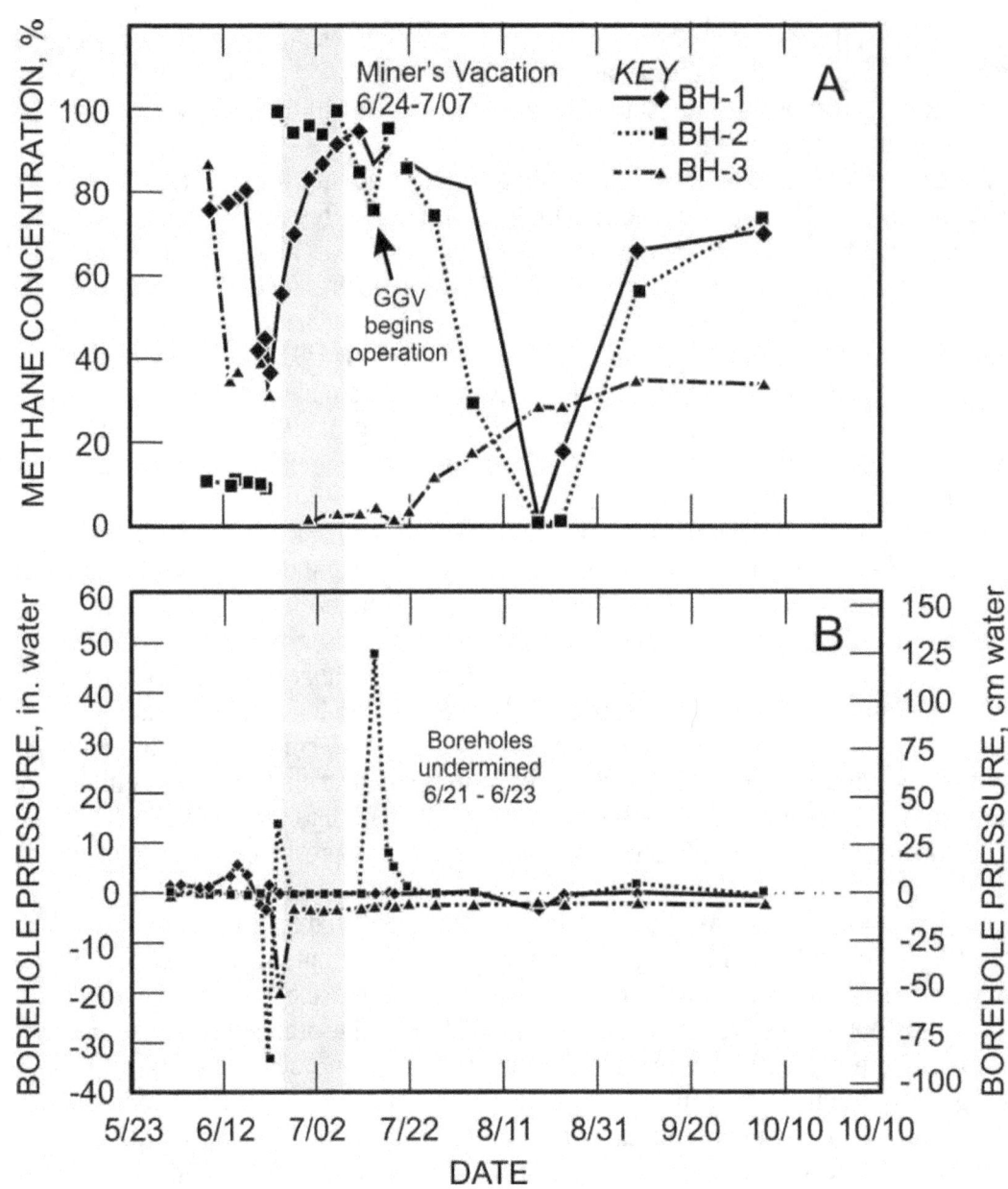

Figure 34.—Methane concentration (A) and static shut-in pressures (B) measured in the boreholes during progress of mining.

Downhole pressure and methane concentration data suggest that experimental boreholes 1 and 2 (32 and 22 m (100 and 72 ft)), respectively, above the mined coalbed) interact and behave similarly to overburden conditions. Borehole 3 (7.3 m (24 ft) above the mined coalbed) responds to mine ventilation pressure, and later to gob pressure conditions.

Summary

- The GGV fracture network can form 24–46 m (80–150 ft) ahead of the mining face. This distance may vary when conventional GGV slotted pipe configurations are used. Much shorter lengths were used during monitoring.

- The loss of water from GGVs can be rapid—from about 32 to 22 m (100 to 22 ft) above the mined coalbed. The rate of water loss was not related to borehole depth.

- Overburden permeabilities within the same overburden test zones were in the ~1-md range prior to undermining and increased to about 100–500 times following undermining, with higher instantaneous peaks.

- The biggest increase in permeability occurred when the longwall face reached the monitoring locations.

- The borehole test interval within the fractured rock responded to overburden gas pressure, and the test interval in the caved zone responded to mine ventilation conditions.

PRACTICAL GUIDELINES FOR CONTROLLING LONGWALL COALBED METHANE

The following practical guidelines are recommended for controlling longwall coalbed methane. All predictions are based on determinations made for the Pittsburgh Coalbed in southwestern Pennsylvania. The senior authors may be contacted at the NIOSH Pittsburgh Research Laboratory for specific cases and application of the methods described.

- It is recommended to use shielding degasification boreholes to decrease emission rates by at least 25% for development entries. Drill these boreholes as close as practically possible (~27 m (90 ft)) to the entries and operate them for at least 6 months to achieve a 25%–50% decrease in emission rates (Section 1).

- Equations for predicting methane emission rates into development entries are presented in Table 3 (Section 1). These relationships assume a supercritical longwall panel developed in the Pittsburgh Coalbed.

- For panel widths greater than 305 m (1,000 ft), a trilateral borehole configuration is recommended for effective draining of methane (Figure 9B). Short across-panel holes at close spacing can also be effective at degassing a panel, but not at shielding development entries (Figure 9D). The required number of holes will depend on seam anisotropic reservoir conditions, but at least 12 holes for a 3,400-m (11,000-ft) long panel are recommended to achieve the same degasification as the trilateral configuration (Section 2).

- If less than 12 months is available for premining gas drainage, degasification should be continued until the borehole is approached by mining. This approach maximizes the quantity of removed methane and reduces methane emission rates (Section 2).

- To avoid shearer coal production delays, it is recommended that continuous GGV production be assured while GGVs are within about 500 ft of the working face. In many mines, the quantity of coalbed methane removed by a GGV is significant, potentially 75% of the volume of gas emissions on the longwall face. A similar finding was observed by prior NIOSH research [Mucho et al. 2000] based on tracer gas injection. If an operating GGV stops producing gas, the gas that was being removed will enter the ventilation system (Section 3).

- Assuming a well-caved gob, increasing the longwall face length by X% will increase the rate of methane emissions by, at most, two-thirds of X%. For example, based on Pittsburgh Seam experimental data, an increase in longwall face length of 25% will increase methane emissions rates by (2/3) × (25%), or 17% (Section 4).

- The length of the slotted casing section of a GGV will strongly influence its level of gas production. To effectively design the slotted casing section of a GGV, it is recommended to:
  - Review the local geology to identify the locations of gas-bearing strata; and
  - Set the top of the slotted section at the highest gas-producing stratigraphic horizon (Section 6).

- Completing a GGV into the caved zone is counterproductive (Figures 24–25) and increases the likelihood of intermittent production from increased-width, supercritical panels. Therefore, the drilling or completion depth of GGVs should be at least 14 m (45 ft) above the mined coalbed for longwall panels, particularly in the Northern Appalachian Basin. This assumes that the caving zone is six to nine times the seam height and production of coalbed gas from the GGV is dominated by the overlying and underlying coalbeds (Sections 6 and 7).

- It is recommended that operators emphasize continuous GGV production since it will potentially produce 40%–50% more coalbed gas than GGVs operating intermittently (Section 7).

- Increasing the longwall panel width increases the quantity of methane present because of the increased fractured reservoir volume. However, this increase does not enhance the performance of GGVs. As panel width increases, the effectiveness of GGVs completed near the tailgate margin will not extend as close to the headgate side. Drilling GGVs on the headgate side or near the panel centerline can produce coalbed gas from this portion of the panel. It is estimated that the central compressed portion of the gob has about one-tenth of the permeability found near the gate road tensional stress zone (Sections 5 and 7).

- In favorable cases, GGVs drilled on the headgate side can be effective. Completion depths must isolate the borehole from communication with the ventilation network (Figure 28). These findings are based on supercritical panel designs (Section 7).

- Mining-induced fracturing was observed to occur 24–46 m (80–150 ft) ahead of the mine face. Boreholes and exhausters should be installed before this occurs (Section 8).

- Data were reviewed for GGV configurations completed from 7 to 32 m (24 to 106 ft) above the mined coalbed for supercritical panels in the Northern Appalachian Basin. It is recommended that GGVs be completed toward the top of this interval and be designed to include the Sewickley Coalbed. Permeabilities overlying the Pittsburgh Coalbed before undermining were very low. Increases in permeability were dramatic following undermining, with increases of about 100–500 times the premining values and instantaneous increases of up to about 1,000 times these values. These measurements did not differ significantly despite differences in boreholes configurations. Fracture permeability pathways remain high to the mined coalbed toward the top of the described interval, yet the likelihood of drawing ventilation air into the borehole is minimized. The post-undermining borehole pressure data also support this finding (Section 8).

REFERENCES

Aul GN, Ray R [1991]. Optimizing methane drainage systems to reduce mine ventilation requirements. In: Proceedings of the Fifth U.S. Mine Ventilation Symposium (Morgantown, WV, June 3–5, 1991).

Bai M, Elsworth D [1993]. Influence of mining geometry on mine hydro-geo-mechanics. SME preprint 93–6. Littleton, CO: Society for Mining, Metallurgy, and Exploration, Inc.

Balusu R, Deguchi G, Holland R, Moreby R, Xue S, Wendt M, Mallet C [2001]. Goaf gas flow mechanics and development of gas and sponcom control strategies at a highly gassy coal mine. In: Proceedings of the Australia-Japan Technology Exchange Workshop (Hunter Valley, Australia, December 2–4, 2001).

Booth CJ, Spande ED [1992]. Potentiometric and aquifer property changes above subsiding longwall mine panels, Illinois basin coalfield. Ground Water $30(2)$:362–368.

Brunner DJ, Schwoebel JJ, Li J [1997]. Simulation based degasification system design for the Shihao mine of the Songzao coal mining administration in Sichuan, China. In: Proceedings of the Sixth International Mine Ventilation Congress (Pittsburgh, PA, May 17–22, 1997).

Brutcher DF, Mehnert BB, van Roosendal DJ, Bauer RA [1990]. Rock strength and overburden changes due to subsidence over a longwall coal mining operation in Illinois. In: Rock Mechanics Contributions and Challenges. Proceedings of the 31st U.S. Symposium on Rock Mechanics (Golden, CO), pp. 563–570.

Cervik J, Fields HH, Aul GN [1975]. Rotary drilling holes in coalbeds for degasification. Pittsburgh, PA: U.S. Department of the Interior, Bureau of Mines, RI 8097. NTIS No. PB 250 693.

Computer Modelling Group [2003]. Generalized equation of state model-GEM: user's guide. Calgary, Alberta, Canada: Computer Modelling Group Ltd.

Curl SJ [1978]. Methane prediction in coal mines. IEA Coal Resources Report ICTIS/TR 04.

Dawson KJ, Istok JD [1991]. Aquifer testing: design and analysis of pumping and slug tests. Chelsea, MI: Lewis Publishers, Inc.

Diamond WP [1994]. Methane control for underground coal mines. Pittsburgh, PA: U.S. Department of the Interior, Bureau of Mines, IC 9395.

Diamond WP, Garcia F [1999]. Prediction of longwall methane emissions: an evaluation of the influence of mining practices on gas emissions and methane control systems. Pittsburgh, PA: U.S. Department of Health and Human Services, Public Health Service, Centers for Disease Control and Prevention, National Institute for Occupational Safety and Health, DHHS (NIOSH) Publication No. 99–150, RI 9649.

Diamond WP, Jeran PW, Trevits MA [1994]. Evaluation of alternative placement of longwall gob gas ventholes for optimum performance. Pittsburgh, PA: U.S. Department of the Interior, Bureau of Mines, RI 9500.

DuBois GM, Kravitz SJ, Reilly JM, Mucho TP [2006]. Target Drilling's long boreholes maximize longwall dimensions. In: Mutmansky JM, Ramani RV, eds. Proceedings of the 11th U.S./North American Mine Ventilation Symposium (University Park, PA, June 5–7, 2006). London: Taylor & Francis Group.

Ertekin T, Sung W, Schwerer FC [1988]. Production performance analysis of horizontal drainage wells for the degasification of coal seams. J Petroleum Technol 40:625–631.

Esterhuizen GS, Karacan CÖ [2005]. Development of numerical models to investigate permeability changes and gas emissions around longwall mining panels. In: Chen G, Huang S, Zhou W, Tinucci J, eds. Proceedings of the 40th U.S. Rock Mechanics Symposium (Anchorage, AK, June 25–29, 2005). Alexandria, VA: American Rock Mechanics Association, pp. 1–13.

Esterhuizen GS, Karacan CÖ [2007]. A methodology for determining gob permeability distributions and its application to reservoir modeling of coal mine longwalls. SME preprint 07–078. Littleton, CO: Society for Mining, Metallurgy, and Exploration, Inc.

Hasenfus GJ, Johnson KL, Su DHW [1988]. A hydrogeomechanical study of overburden aquifer response to longwall mining. In: Proceedings of the Seventh International Conference on Ground Control in Mining. Morgantown, WV: West Virginia University, pp. 149–162.

Hoek E, Bray JW [1981]. Rock slope engineering. 3rd ed. London: Institute of Mining and Metallurgy.

Itasca Consulting Group [2000]. Fast Lagrangian analysis of continua. 2nd ed. Minneapolis, MN: Itasca Consulting Group, Inc.

Itasca Consulting Group [2005]. FLAC3D user's guide. Version 3.0. Minneapolis, MN: Itasca Consulting Group, Inc.

Karacan CÖ [forthcoming]. Evaluation of the relative importance of coalbed reservoir parameters for prediction of methane inflow rates during mining of longwall development entries. Computers & Geosciences.

Karacan CÖ, Diamond WP, Esterhuizen GS, Schatzel SJ [2005]. Numerical analysis of the impact of longwall panel width on methane emissions and performance of gob gas ventholes. In: Proceedings of the International Coalbed Methane Symposium (May 18–19, 2005). Tuscaloosa, AL: University of Alabama, pp. 1–28.

Karacan CÖ, Diamond WP, Schatzel SJ, Garcia F [2006]. Development and application of reservoir models for the evaluation and optimization of longwall methane control systems. In: Mutmansky JM, Ramani RV, eds. Proceedings of the 11th U.S./North American Mine Ventilation Symposium (University Park, PA, June 5–7, 2006). London: Taylor & Francis Group, pp. 425–432.

Karacan CÖ, Diamond WP, Schatzel SJ [2007a]. Numerical analysis of the influence of in-seam horizontal methane drainage boreholes on longwall face emission rates. Int J Coal Geol 72(1):15–32.

Karacan CÖ, Esterhuizen GS, Schatzel SJ, Diamond WP [2007b]. Reservoir simulation-based modeling for characterizing longwall methane emissions and gob gas venthole production. Int J Coal Geol 71(2–3):225–245.

King GR, Ertekin T, Schwerer FC [1986]. Numerical simulation of the transient behavior of coal-seam degasification wells. Society of Petroleum Engineers (SPE) Formation Evaluation. April, pp. 165–183.

Kolesar J, Ertekin T [1986]. The unsteady state nature of sorption and diffusion phenomena in the micropore structure of coal. In: Proceedings of the Society of Petroleum Engineers (SPE) Unconventional Gas Technology Symposium (Louisville, KY). Paper No. 15233, pp. 289–314.

Krog RB, Schatzel SJ, Garcia F, Marshall JK [2006]. Predicting methane emissions from longer longwall faces by analysis of emission contributors. In: Mutmansky JM, Ramani RV, eds. Proceedings of the 11th U.S./North American Mine Ventilation Symposium (University Park, PA, June 5–7, 2006). London: Taylor & Francis Group, pp. 383–392.

Louis C [1969]. A study of groundwater flow in jointed rock and its influence on the stability of rock masses [Dissertation]. University of Karlsruhe, Germany.

Matetic RJ, Liu J, Elsworth D [1995]. Using multiple-point borehole extensometers and finite-element modeling in coordination with hydrologic field data to determine postmining effects to the ground water system. Presented at the Outdoor Action Conference, National Ground Water Association (Las Vegas, NV, May 2–9, 1995).

McCulloch CM, Diamond WP, Bench BM, Deul M [1975]. Selected geological factors affecting mining of the Pittsburgh coalbed. Pittsburgh, PA: U.S. Department of the Interior, RI 8093. NTIS No. PB 249 851.

Mucho TP, Diamond WP, Garcia F, Byars JD, Cario SL [2000]. Implications of recent NIOSH tracer gas studies on bleeder and gob gas ventilation design. SME preprint 00–8. Littleton, CO: Society for Mining, Metallurgy, and Exploration, Inc.

Munson DE, Nenzley SE [1980]. Analytic subsidence model using void-volume distribution functions. In: Proceedings of the 21st U.S. Rock Mechanics Symposium (Rolla, MO).

Noack K [1998]. Control of gas emissions in underground coal mines. Int J Coal Geol *35*(1–4):57–82.

Palchik V [2003]. Formation of fractured zones in overburden due to longwall mining. Environ Geol *44*(1):28–38.

Pappas DM, Mark C [1993]. Behavior of simulated gob material. Pittsburgh, PA: U.S. Department of the Interior, Bureau of Mines, RI 9458.

Peng SS, Chiang HS [1984]. Longwall mining. New York: Wiley.

Remner DJ, Ertekin T, Sung W, King GR [1986]. A parametric study of the effects of coal seam properties on gas drainage efficiency. SPE Reservoir Eng *Nov*:633–645.

Schatzel SJ, Garcia F, McCall FE [1992]. Methane sources and emissions on two longwall panels of a Virginia coal mine. In: Proceedings of the Ninth Annual International Pittsburgh Coal Conference (Pittsburgh, PA, October 12–16, 1992), pp. 991–998.

Schatzel SJ, Krog RB, Garcia F, Marshall JK, Trackemas J [2006]. Prediction of longwall methane emissions and the associated consequences of increasing longwall face lengths: a case study in the Pittsburgh coalbed. In: Mutmansky JM, Ramani RV, eds. Proceedings of the 11th U.S./North American Mine Ventilation Symposium (University Park, PA, June 5–7, 2006). London: Taylor & Francis Group, pp. 375–382.

Singh MM, Kendorski FS [1981]. Strata disturbance prediction for mining beneath surface water and waste impoundments. In: Proceedings of the First Conference on Ground Control in Mining. Morgantown, WV: West Virginia University, pp. 76–89.

Smith AC, Diamond WP, Mucho TP, Organiscak JA [1994]. Bleederless ventilation systems as a spontaneous combustion control measure in U.S. coal mines. Pittsburgh, PA: U.S. Department of the Interior, Bureau of Mines, IC 9377. NTIS No. PB 94–152816.

Smith DM, Williams FL [1984]. Diffusional effects in the recovery of methane from coalbeds. SPE J *Oct*:529–535.

Spencer SJ, Somers ML, Pinchewski WV, Doig ID [1987]. Numerical simulation of gas drainage from coal seams. In: Proceedings of the 62nd Society of Petroleum Engineers (SPE) Annual Technical Conference and Exhibition. Paper No. 16857, pp. 217–229.

Stephenson D [1979]. Rockfill in hydraulic engineering. Amsterdam, Netherlands: Elsevier.

Tauziede C, Pokryszka Z, Carrau A, Saraux E [1997]. Modeling of gas circulation in the goaf of retreat faces. In: Proceedings of the Sixth International Mine Ventilation Congress (Pittsburgh, PA, May 17–22, 1997).

Thakur PC [1981]. Methane control for longwall gobs. In Ramani RV, ed. Longwall-shortwall mining: state of the art. New York: Society of Mining Engineers, pp. 81–86.

Thakur PC [2006]. Coal seam degasification. In: Kissell FN, ed. Handbook for methane control in mining. Pittsburgh, PA: U.S. Department of Health and Human Services, Public Health Service, Centers for Disease Control and Prevention, National Institute for Occupational Safety and Health, DHHS (NIOSH) Publication No. 2006–127, IC 9486, pp. 77–96.

Thakur PC, Poundstone WN [1980]. Horizontal drilling technology for advance degasification. Min Eng *Jun:*676–680.

Wendt M, Balusu R [2001]. CFD modeling of longwall goaf gas flow dynamics. In: Proceedings of the Australia-Japan Technology Exchange Workshop (Hunter Valley, Australia, December 2–4, 2001).

Young GBC [1998]. Computer modeling and simulation of coalbed methane resources. Int J Coal Geol *35*(1–4):369–379.

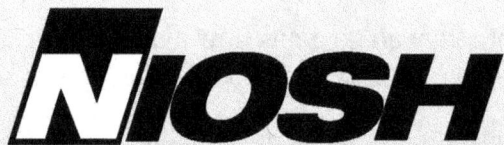

Delivering on the Nation's promise:
safety and health at work for all people
through research and prevention

To receive NIOSH documents or more information about occupational safety and health topics, contact NIOSH at

1–800–CDC–INFO (1–800–232–4636)
TTY: 1–888–232–6348
e-mail: cdcinfo@cdc.gov

or visit the NIOSH Web site at **www.cdc.gov/niosh.**

For a monthly update on news at NIOSH, subscribe to NIOSH *eNews* by visiting **www.cdc.gov/niosh/eNews.**

DHHS (NIOSH) Publication No. 2008–114

SAFER • HEALTHIER • PEOPLE™